Ontologies and Natures

Ontologies and Natures

Knowledge about Health in Visual Culture

Milton Fernando Gonzalez Rodriguez

LEXINGTON BOOKS
Lanham • Boulder • New York • London

Published by Lexington Books
An imprint of The Rowman & Littlefield Publishing Group, Inc.
4501 Forbes Boulevard, Suite 200, Lanham, Maryland 20706
www.rowman.com

86-90 Paul Street, London EC2A 4NE

British Library Cataloguing in Publication Information Available

Library of Congress Cataloging-in-Publication Data

Names: Gonzalez Rodriguez, Milton Fernando, author.
Title: Ontologies and natures : knowledge about health in visual culture / Milton Fernando Gonzalez Rodriguez.
Description: Lanham, Maryland : Lexington Books, [2023] | Includes bibliographical references and index.
Identifiers: LCCN 2022031388 (print) | LCCN 2022031389 (ebook) | ISBN 9781666909494 (cloth) | ISBN 9781666909500 (ebook) Subjects:
LCSH: Communication in public health. | Visual communication in science. | Nature, Healing power of. | Health in mass media. | Social medicine.
Classification: LCC RA423.2 .G66 2023 (print) | LCC RA423.2 (ebook) | DDC 362.101/4—dc23/eng/20220722
LC record available at https://lccn.loc.gov/2022031388
LC ebook record available at https://lccn.loc.gov/2022031389

Contents

Acknowledgments

I dedicate this book to my mother, María Melba Rodriguez de Gonzalez, who taught me in her own way that knowing and (re)searching are intrinsically related. One depends on the other. As much as I have also depended on the hundreds of intellectual exchanges I have had with Martin Karl Andersen on the contents of this book. He has been there during the most challenging moments and this monograph owes its existence to him, as much as to me. Mange tak! In like manner, I thank Eric, Leo, Bibi, Paul, Nando, Irene, Francesca, Phil, Ana, Xiao, and Tintin for not giving up on me, despite the reduced attention and time I could devote to them while writing this book.

Heartfully, I want to thank all those who have taken the time to provide help in one way or another. Along the path, I have received encouragement, advice, feedback, and support from scholars to whom I will always be indebted. Special thanks goes to Kaat Wils for everything she has done for me. Her disposition, enthusiasm, and engagement were the starting point of the Marie Skłodowska-Curie Individual Fellowship that allowed me to complete this book as a fellow at KU Leuven. Her support and feedback were crucial during the revision stage and many parts of the revised version benefited from her immense knowledge in the history of medicine. At Leuven, I want to specially thank all the members of the Cultural History since 1750 Research Group for their collegiality, support, kindness, and friendship. It has been wonderful to be part of such an inspiring, talented, and friendly team. KU Leuven has truly changed my perception of what university community means and I am very proud of being able to do research in such a stimulating environment.

In similar ways, I want to express my gratitude to Dániel Margócsy, for his support and for being, as someone called him once, "one the most knowledgeable, dedicated, coolest and nicest historians." I thank him for his feedback, intellectual generosity, and for sharing with me some of his incredible knowledge about visual culture and history. At Cambridge, I also want to thank Françoise Barbira Freedman, Mary Augusta Brazelton, and Simon Schaffer for sharing their expertise on specific sources. I cannot thank enough the Department of History and Philosophy of Science at the University of Cambridge for hosting me as a visiting scholar and allowing me to use its resources during important writing and revision stages of this book. I want to specially thank Raphaëlle Goyeau and Jack Dixon for their help with the Whipple Library book collection, for their prompt and timely advice. No writing in the UK would have been possible without a roof over my head. Hence, I want to express my appreciation to Clare Hall College for housing me during the long, dark, and stormy evenings while I was revising and redrafting the manuscript.

Furthermore, I owe also special thanks to Prof. Thomas Gaslonde at the Musée François Tillequin/Paris Descartes University and Prof. Steffen Sammler at the Leibniz Institute for Educational Media | Georg Eckert Institute for their time, expertise, and support. At Lexington, I want to specially thank Kasey Beduhn, Courtney Morales, Emma Ebert, Mark Lopez, Jayanthi Chander and Deanta Global for their efficiency and encouragement. I take this opportunity also to extend my gratitude to the anonymous reviewers for accepting the task of reading the manuscript, showing their willingness to share their expertise, and providing useful feedback that could be used to improve the revised final version. A special thanks goes also to Íþrótta- og ólympíusamband Íslands/The National Olympic and Sports Association of Iceland for allowing me to use their campaign's poster image.

Finally, I wish, above all, to acknowledge my profound gratitude to people from all corners of the globe, from Kyrgyzstan to Mexico, who helped me in one way or another to complete this book project. Some of them facilitated my access to historical sources, others showed me the way around museums, or answered my questions in stores and factories. A couple corrected me about misunderstandings concerning the origin of raw materials or provided advice about digital sources unknown to me. Some anonymous informants directed my attention to important details in the visual surfaces and artifacts discussed in this book, and I cannot thank all of them enough for their generosity and time.

This book project has received funding from the European Union's Horizon 2020 research and innovation program under the Marie Skłodowska-Curie grant agreement No 101026198, for which I am honored and humbled.

Introduction

Ontologies, Bioclusivity, and Epistemic Semiotics

Societies use visual cultural production differently to express their understanding about nature and its healing properties. Human experience is layered with and conditioned by the jagged intensities caused by disease at various stages, either temporarily or permanently. By default, being free of illness and injury defines the quality of the time we spend on this planet. Yet, the perception of nature as a healing source, and its representation, varies considerably. Images implicitly become cultural sites that distinctly reflect how their creators ontologically perceive and relate to their surroundings. In this sense, visual surfaces can provide, on the one hand, information about the ways in which their makers imagine, understand and deploy nature as part of their own health-preventing, -enhancing, and -restoring practices. On the other hand, they can also operate as venues where individuals and societies articulate their impressions about others' therapeutic practices and medicinal knowledge. In both cases, the visual realm encapsulates some of the ideas we have about the relationship between epistemologies, health, and the natural world. A set of interdependencies that eventually materialize in cultural outputs. If we pay attention, I argue, references to the care and cure of the body can be found everywhere. With that premise in mind, this book considers how, for instance, a YouTube vlog, a film, a toy, a teabag, natural products packaging (figure 0.1), an infographic, an antiwrinkle cream, footage of a lake, and a cannabis cigarette can be considered as part of the visual history and present of health and knowledge. The ubiquitousness of medicine as a

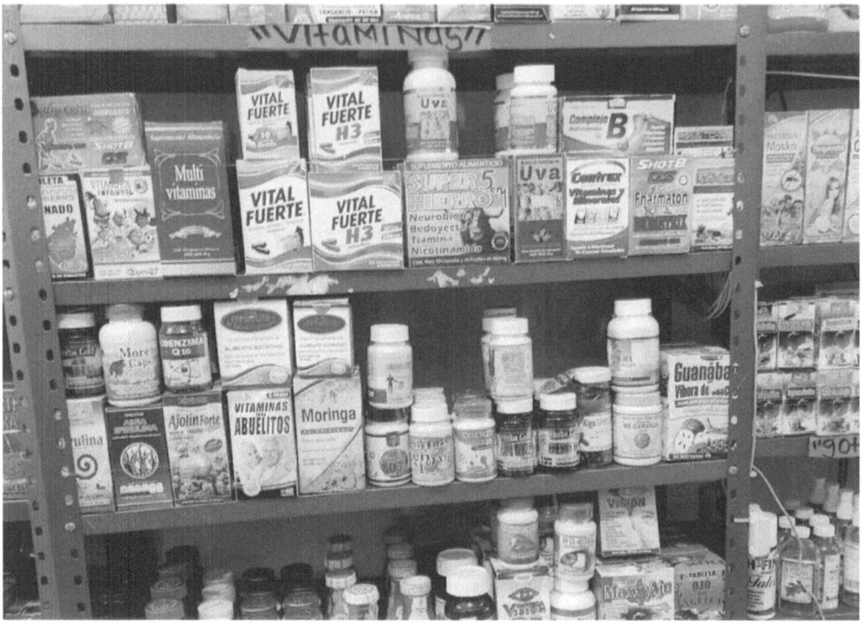

Figure 0.1 Shelf in a Natural Product Store in the State of Oaxaca, Mexico. *Source*: Photo by author.

theme explains the diversity of the corpus of the book in terms of format, shape, genre, content, composition, and, in the case of psychotropic substances, relative intangibility. A commonality shared by all of the selected objects of study is that their characterization is contextualized through the lens of naturality (the state of being natural or related to nature). Ergo, the present volume delves into the ways in which images register the relation between social groups and their health epistemic ecosystems, or those of others.

From a theoretical perspective, the selected study cases are intended to show examples of *epistemology of the familiar*, defined by Rentetzi (2020) as "the study of the ordinary, the ephemeral, and the often unnoticed" (38). The discussions in the subsequent chapters advance the idea that seemingly trivial objects and practices are, regardless of their presumed insubstantiality, reflections of episteme-informed attitudes and assumptions. I argue that ordinary visual surfaces (e.g., a colorful toy test tube), despite their unremarkableness, operate as epistemic sites, not because they pursue to disseminate knowledge, but because there is *a* type of knowledge behind their creation.[1] In Platonian terms, the goal (*ergon*) of representations about medicinal knowledge may not indeed per se be to inform about the epistemes, doxa, or techne that underpin the preservation and restoration of health. Yet, since images and visual surfaces are at their core meaning-producing sites, they operate as input and output about the epistemic systems where they emerge. After all, "mundane objects" also play a role in the "emergence of new structures of knowledge" (38).

From a methodological viewpoint, the book is informed by historical sources, visual and virtual ethnography, content analysis, and semiotic-linguistic analysis. As a theme, the nature-knowledge-health triad is approached from various vantage points within and across the humanities. The interdisciplinary discussion revolves around artifacts and images that have circulated throughout centuries and corners of the world. The book is a preliminary attempt to explore how historical, cultural, ideological, and social intricacies are the backbone of the conventions and conversations that inform the nature-health relation in each group. In an era overtly marked by the excessive presence and use of images, few venues, I posit, can offer better insights into the interplay between societies, their medicinal practices, and the role assigned to nature within their health landscapes. In the case of cultural artifacts informed by Indigenous knowledge(s) (e.g., a documentary), an attempt has been made to abide by Mahuika's (2019) observation that "oral history is not something to be found merely in a recorded interview" (1). Attention is paid to the fact that plurality and specificity imbue the variety of approaches to medicinal practices that communities have evolved across time and space. As I suggest, considering the spectrum encompassed by visual culture provides insights about the multiplicity of epistemic systems at an ontological level. Therefore, as the title suggests, throughout the book, I use the word ontology in plural form, as I believe it articulates more accurately the heterogeneity showcased in the objects of study.

ONTOLOGIES

The definition of ontology varies according to the various schools of philosophy. Levinas's view on the subject (1951) is that function is instrumental as a state category where ontological considerations are reflections of nomenclatures based on the things that occupy space.[2] Using an unsophisticated example to explain his point, this means that, for instance, a spearmint flavored chewing gum ought to be recognized as a categorizable object. The being of the chewing gum is presumably a constituent of purpose-defined domains and systems that depend on the interrelation between them to maintain the dynamic that explains how they are connected. Despite its apparent unremarkableness, the piece of gum exists as it serves a purpose. In Westerhoff's terms (2005), ontology is about focusing on the things that matter the most, inquiring which objects belong to each identified category, and how they relate to, and by extension, exclude and contain one another. In this sense, the chewing gum's flavor, materiality, texture, malleability, and (literal) plasticity inform and confirm its existence and hence, a possible designation within a category and further interrelations. The focus lies then on distinguishing some objects from others while paying attention to the distance, proximity, or interdependence between one another as referents to situate them conceptually. From this viewpoint, the difference and similarities between this particular chewing gum and, for instance, nicotine chewing gum create an ontological relation between the two.

Alternatively, from a fluxist standpoint, pondering about ontology involves reflecting on the processes that define the objects of the world. Being is then the temporality of an object within an event that leads it to realize its purpose.[3] Proceeding with the abovementioned example, for the imagined piece of gum, chewing constitutes the presence of the event that would circumscribe the operationalization of its function.

In terms of pursuit, "Ontology seeks to provide definitive and exhaustive classification of entities in all spheres of being."[4] An aspect that touches particularly upon the subject of visibility and visuality. As I show in this book, images pose ontological challenges in terms of purpose, relatedness, referentiality, and content. While a photograph, for example, of a spearmint plant can be regarded as archival material for an ethnobotanical repository, the picture can also be considered to serve an epistemic purpose (i.e., knowing the spearmint plant exists and what it looks like). The image documents the state of being, but also of knowing (*episteme*). The same photo operates as a vehicle to mobilize a framed representation of the object in question. An awareness that leads to the realization of a different place and temporal dimension in which the object resides or circulates. A background scenario for the existence, in this case, of the photographed spearmint plant, signals the actuality of other objects related or unrelated to the place it occupies (where the picture is taken). Lastly, the intentionality behind the creation of the image is a matter of content. The spearmint plant is central in the optic composition because it conveys meaning, possibly through references, cues, and signs (*sēmeion*), in one way or another. Regardless of their context, visuals provide information and are receptacles of data. They are simultaneously part of an epistemic and semiotic system. Classification of images is therefore a complex process. Perhaps as convoluted as creating categories that properly convey the ontological relations and dependencies that interlink data without reducing them or fragmenting them. Referring back to the spearmint-flavored chewing gum example, the photograph of the spearmint plant and the piece of gum, depending on how one chooses to categorize them (or parts thereof), might be ontologically relatable. Even it's most likely the case that the gum does not actually *contain* or is *made of* spearmint.

Beyond the abstract world of philosophy, the applicability of ontological approaches percolates various domains of human knowledge.[5] The suitability of ontology in environments, such as engineering and informatics, rests on the premise that relations, properties, labels, and categories are preceded by a definition of each one of them.[6] More pertinent in the case of this book, ontological considerations underpin the inscription of biomedicine within systems that require classifications and identifying taxonomies. In biomedical informatics, for instance, it matters how to establish nomenclatures of terminologies[7] and how to associate material with nonmaterial entities (e.g., surfaces).[8] The functionality of ontologies in retrieving information, for example, about specific conditions, genes, tissues, patients, and medical histories, build on creating systems that link knowledge and hermeneutic interfaces.[9]

The versatility of applications of ontology is nevertheless not the reason why I use the term in the plural form throughout the book. I do so departing from the view that objects constitute parts of a system (whole) and that these wholes are related to one another in different ways and taking a diversity of forms. On that account, I agree with Ingarden (1964) about the whole as a superstructure composed of ontological layers that define dependencies between elements, a relation embedded in the history of each one of them and of the whole as a host ecosystem. As for the plural emergence of ontologies, I refer to Poli's (1996) observations about the distinction between the history of a whole (system) and the history of its location, as a result of a shifting composition of the constituting elements and objects, additions, subtractions, and modifications.[10] I suggest that the situatedness of each ontological framework is liable to the acknowledgment and knowledge of those who recognize it as a superstructure of dependencies in each case. The diversity of habitats, interrelations, dependencies, and dynamics between locations and human systems superimposed on those spaces suggest, I argue, that there is not a singular ontology understood as an organizational framework. Smith (2012) points out that ontology "seeks not predication and explanation but rather taxonomy and description" (48). Ontologies in plural can be considered then, I suggest, as the manifold frameworks that recognize that elements enact dependencies across a system, but not necessarily across systems. They are many, not parallel, not comparable, and not singular. They are plural as the nature-health dependencies identified in various forms and contexts in distinct scenarios (images/visual surfaces) across the cases explored in the next chapters. A sense of multiplicity that also seems to apply to the various definitions of health.

(Ecological) Health

Health is difficult to define as it involves establishing parameters for what it means not to have good health, be unhealthy and be ill, and what distinguishes one from the other. For some, health cannot limit itself to biophysical constraints or a scrutinization based primarily on the absence or presence of diseases.[11] In doing so, the term "risks" reducing the domains and areas of human life where the well-being of the body intersects with other cultural and social dimensions not necessarily defined by biomedical rubrics. For Adamson (2019), "Health is a medical concept, indeed, the concept that gives medicine both its definition and its raison d'être" (2). Kingma (2019) demonstrates through examples taken from the history of attitudes toward homosexuality and nuanced ways of thinking of blindness that an attempt of defining health involves, almost unavoidably, a review of dominant values about what is considered to be healthy and unhealthy. In her words, "To make progress in these debates, we need to ask not *whether* values play a role but *how* they do so, and *which* values are important" (317) (author's own emphasis). In normativist terms, health and its absence, presumably marked by the presence of disease, are states described through value-laden conceptualizations. Sometimes presented in contrast with naturalist views, normativism regards culture as a decisive element in acknowledged understandings of what it entails to be ill. Normativism and naturalism are not necessarily opposing views but a naturalist standpoint regards objective biological facts as premises to define when someone is sick, disease-free, or finds herself in a continuum between these two conditions. The debate in philosophy of medicine includes nuanced postulations underpinned by other approaches as well.[12] After all, "Medicine generates some of the most powerful vehicles for disapproval and approbation, for expressing moral values in naturalized forms."[13]

For Leonardi (2018), health "may be conceptualized as the capability to react to all kinds of environmental events having the desired emotional, cognitive, and behavioral responses and avoiding those undesirable ones" (742). This definition seems to accommodate the various dimensions that the bodily experience cocoons throughout domains that include also nonbiomedical determinants in the strict sense of the word. An assessment of degrees of desirability remains nevertheless problematic as it is perhaps not always clear where the qualifiers "desired" and "undesired" begin or/and end. In like manner, it might not be possible to pinpoint exactly where the boundaries of the "emotional" realm are and what constitutes an emotion. Leonardi's conceptualization expands in any case the horizon of what health entails by including actualizations that underscore more global understandings of the role of the human mind in physical well-being. Since reacting and responding precede the adoption of behaviors, emphasis is placed on the agency of those who pursuit health. They are the actors and performers in the promotion and creation of optimal "environmental events." The desired and undesired outcomes depend on it.

While environment in this context does not explicitly refer to what Schemmel (2020) identifies as "planetary ecological system" (7), no life on the planet, and hence no health landscapes can realistically thrive in the twenty-first century without implementing long-term policies of restoration, preservation, mitigation, and damage control of ecosystems. Environmental matters are matters of survival and by proxy, of life and death. Isolation in rural areas of Madagascar, inhospitable climatic abruptness in Siberia, and altitude across the Andes, for instance, are all factors that have defined how local societies have developed mechanisms to cope with their immediate surroundings. As Hamati-Ataya (2022) notes, "from their original Afrotropical context of emergence," humankind's globalization "has been achieved through journeys taken, with varying degrees of risk and success, across the earth's biogeographically patterned canvas—along its corridors, around its barriers, and via its refugia" (14). Learning to know the new environments has been crucial for societies to provide food and shelter, and logically also to treat disease. But what happens when our ecosystems dramatically change?

The process of conscientization at a global level about the gravity of the matter has prompted responses at a micro- and macro-level context. The human need to record and express visual reactions to experiences has materialized in millions (perhaps billions) of visual cultural artifacts that have registered the evolution, development, and impact of the current environmental catastrophe. In addition to the expected marked presence of societies traditionally active in the use of communicational channels, easily overlooked communities are finding in visual media formats a platform to voice their concerns and share their points of view (e.g., Indigenous peoples).[14] Perhaps by force of circumstance, we live in a time where visual culture outlets are becoming inter-epistemological stages of mediation and exchange. Moved by spaces created at the interstices of interconnected networks of media production, today more than ever before, there are plenty of opportunities and possibilities to find out how each of us relates to the natural world, how our communities regard the planet, and how we think we will survive climate change and global warming.

While, for instance, the Embera community (Colombia) collectively places emphasis on documenting their cosmologies and ethnobotanical heritage in *Jaibaná Bedea* (2015), director Jari Kokko follows the lives of Finns affected by mold sickness in *Kanarialinnut* (2015), and Dorn Bouttasing explores the interdependence between riverscapes and beinghood in *Lives of the Ou River* (Laos, 2010).[15] The diversity of approaches to the human body in the context of ecological paradigms, disease, medicinal knowledge, and survival attests to particular elements of geographical location, epistemic systems, and conceptualization of what health means. Each of these distinct societies and their components experience, perceive, regard, and act toward nature differently. Not only because they obviously inhabit ecosystems structured and surrounded in dissimilar manners. Their accumulated experiences, knowledge systems, and beliefs differ as much as the flora, fauna, and specificities of their ecospheres.

Schemmel (2020) alerts us about the universality of knowledge and science production and the importance of this realization in the face of an environmental crisis. I argue that the most challenging aspect of the nature-knowledge-health triad in ecological terms is that each society has its own understanding of how it ought to relate to the environment it inhabits, and how this relationship determines its well-being. As I suggest throughout the book, each community interacts with its surroundings on its own terms, adhering to protocols and interdependencies only its members understand and which I define as *bioclusivity.*

Bioclusivity

A biodiverse world logically implies there is a wide array of ways in which large and small societies cohabit, adapt, reshape, and perceive the realm of living organisms and processes that encompass life on Earth. Presumably, one of the commonalities members of social groups share is a cumulative set of ideas about nature according to the attitudes prevailing in each community, and that only in-group individuals recognize and comprehend. Those who not are conversant or familiar with the dominant ontological framework are outsiders. They are not the addressees of conversations held at the core of communities of which they are not part. In this sense, a separation is made between "inclusive we" and "exclusive we." I suggest that this marked distinction, known in linguistics as clusivity, can be useful to articulate ontological and epistemological differences. Since we all have profoundly dystonic views about nature and life (*bios*) on this planet, it seems normal that this hampers our mutual understanding. Throughout this book, I use the term *bioclusivity* to refer to the worldview held by the members of a specific group about nature, and which dwells in the interstices of what makes each culture unique. In light of the importance of health for all humans, I argue that a sense of bioclusivity filters and informs our approach to the care and cure of the body. This is because similar practices, overlapping epistemologies, and diffusion of more dominant epistemic systems have not yet erased or eroded the specific relation some societies share with their home environments. Their inclusion-exclusion distinction is clear. Conflict emerges from having different bioclusivity protocols, typified, for instance, by the tensions between Indigenous societies in the Amazon and Western mining companies.

It is through shared common experiences, cohabitation, daily interaction, intergenerational legacy, and formal and informal educational settings that we as individuals internalize the relation with the natural world that aligns with the one acknowledged by our native communities. Bioclusivity, I argue, is part of the social mindset of a society. It is a matter of how naturality evokes and invokes a particular sets of beliefs, practices, attitudes, perspectives, outlooks, inclinations, and standpoints.[16] This agreement is tacit and goes beyond having different opinions or political views. Embracing a particular way of experiencing nature, I posit, is part of our socialization process. There is probably no society void of traditions, norms, principles, rules, or policies on how to negotiate or force their presence in the landscapes they occupy. The physical areas settled by a community become the *mise-en-scene* where the human-nature interaction takes place. The actors have an idea of what their role is and are aware of what lies within the boundaries of the scenario where their presence unfolds. Geographical, climatological, biological, hydrological, and environmental conditions determine to a large extent human lifestyles and have done for thousands of years. After all, "environmental knowledges that enabled human communities to exploit the landscape, its connective features, and the biotic world it contained," presumably emerged as part of the "epistemic apparatus" first developed during the Paleolithic (Hamati-Ataya, 2022, 3). Our tools have emerged as tangible strategies primarily for survival and as mechanisms to navigate the physicality of the spaces where we dwell or to search for new frontiers or routines. Accumulation of experiences through knowledge and development of techniques and technologies have endowed us with the capacity to understand what to expect from the geographical spaces that surround us (and in some cases, those further afield).

At the core, the conversation revolves around the symbiotic interplay between human life, nature, and health. Ecological concerns are health concerns. Coronavirus, climate change, and global warming are intrinsically linked to the interaction between humans and ecosystems. Looking at the present situation, terrestrial and marine habitats depend more than ever, on the self-appointed managers- and administrators-of-nature role taken up by humans. A call for environmental awareness has made more visible the diversity of attitudes toward nature across hemispheres and oceans. Not all cultures interact with nature in the same way and they do not routinely have discussions on how to go about it. As I see it, each society dwells in its own bioclusivity, circumlocutorily agreed upon between its members. There are multiple examples of the determinative role of culture in the projects of harnessing resources, compartmentalization of green areas, (over)consumption of nonorganic goods that risk becoming unnecessary waste, acceptable and unacceptable sources of energy, and use of technology in a(n) (un)sustainable fashion. Economic interests have distinguished the deployment of policies where profits are prioritized over long-term ecological considerations.

The world is still divided according to rubrics dictated by wealth, political influence, military power, and operationalization of knowledge. The problematic aspect of the current climate crisis, just as the COVID-19 pandemic, is that, although they seem to affect some more than others, their implications will take a toll on everyone living on this planet. As Renn (2020) asserts, "developed countries may actually appear to benefit from climate change, while developing countries suffer—but ultimately everyone will lose. There will be no escape, not even for the rich" (4). The awareness of this unavoidable fact has prompted nations to discuss possible scenarios, but compromises are difficult to reach in light of possible economic losses. Communities living in fragile habitats risk bearing the brunt of rising oceans and temperatures. Their survival depends on reaching an agreement and consensus. Yet, as I suggest, the conundrum lies in the impossibility of nations of reflecting on the orders, nomenclatures, and regimes (bioclusivity) that have informed their relation with nature for decades and centuries (millennia in some cases). Relatively fixed within a mindset that only insiders understand, the clusivity aspect prevails over the *bios* aspect, leading to debates with no satisfactory outcome.

Avoiding essentialist views, the fact remains that many societies regard nature as their primary source of well-being. They seem to see a direct correlation between preservation of ecosystems and the right balance needed to keep communities healthy. Defined by their own genesis as nations, in stark contrast, the synergies at play are quite different in larger urban hubs or highly advanced economies steered by profit-driven complex networks. The current ecological crisis and its possible remediation depend on reaching an agreement. It is a challenge. We are all conversant in the bioclusivity protocols of the societies where we belong, live, or recognize as our own. This limits our worldviews to the detriment or against the possibility of sharing the same planet without destroying it. If socialization is not necessarily an addendum to the social contract we sign at birth, neither is an invitation to internalize the sense of bioclusivity of one's community. Yet, encounters with nature, as much as social norms, are unavoidable parts of life in a society. Small and large social groups, starting with one's family, pave the road to become conversant in the bioclusivity codes acknowledged by the other members of the community. An important observation about the notion of bioclusivity is that it denotes an ever-evolving set of protocols continuously updated by epistemic exchanges, additions, and transfers, idiosyncratically coupled to each society. A key point to bear in mind is that being exposed to or having an encounter with an image does not mean we are the addressees ("inclusive we" vis-à-vis "exclusive we").

Cultural outputs, such as the examples reviewed in the next section, mirror how specificities and distinctiveness of the nature-knowledge-health triad have evolved across time and space. Notwithstanding, they retain their reportorial value in registering and informing viewers who encounter them about the societies, context, and bioclusivity behind their production.[17]

NATURE, KNOWLEDGE, AND HEALTH IN IMAGES

Nature and visual representations have followed the same path ever since the first humans registered in stone their inherent need to use figurations to express, articulate, or mediate their sense of the world. The 43,900-year-old representations of a warty pig (*Sus celebensis*), such as the ones found in a South Sulawesi cave, contextualize and historicize a passage in the visual autobiography humanity has created through thousands of years.[18] Representing what belongs to the human condition means to locate humans in relation to their surroundings. Visual surfaces are portals to delve into the processes by which an image adds, discards, embellishes, downplays, or champions certain aspects over others. As the next six examples from various moments in history and different corners of the globe show, graphical representations can provide, on the one hand, insights about the role of nature within the creators' epistemic systems and health landscapes. On the other, they can mirror the impressions about knowledge systems and hence medicinal practices

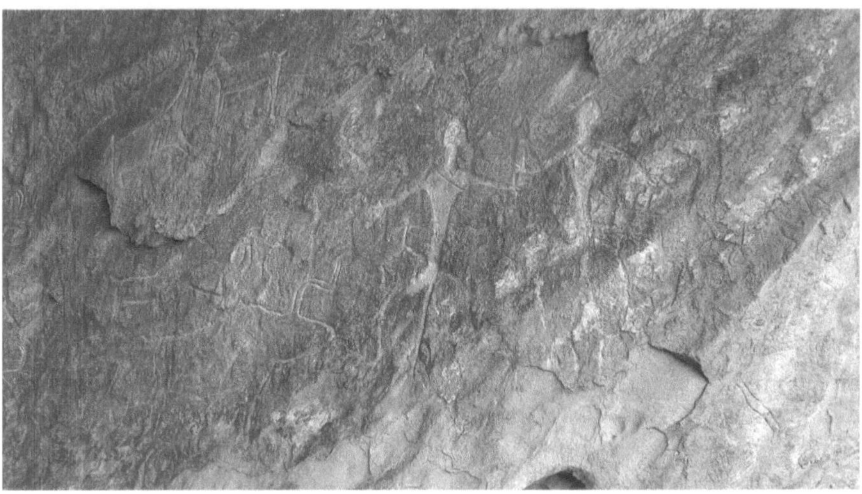

Figure 0.2 One of the ca. 6,000 Petroglyphs Located in Gobustan, Azerbaijan. *Source*: Photo taken by the author during a visit to Qobustan dövlət tarixi-bədii qoruğu (Gobustan State Historical and Cultural Reserve) in 2016.

presumed to be foreign to the society where the image or cultural artifact circulates. In both cases, they facilitate the reproduction of encounters between the moment the image was made and is subsequently seen.

Some of the oldest pictorial representations known to us, in one way or another, make reference to the relation between well-being, environment, and survival. I have therefore chosen as first example (figure 0.2) one of the 6,000 petroglyphs found in the Gobustan Site, located in the eastern part of modern-day Azerbaijan. Since a proposed periodization of the images suggests that Gobustan petroglyphs include images pecked, scratched, or incised between the High Pleistocene and the sixteenth century,[19] this petroglyph exemplifies the capacity of visual surfaces to mediate and register changes in the human-environment relationship over thousands of years.

The environment has obviously changed since the time the earliest petroglyphs were created.[20] The visual representation of boats in an area relatively far away from water prompts questions about the conditions in which some of the authors of the petroglyphs lived or reached the site. Pictorial renderings of, for instance, lions and wild buffalos strengthen the theory that the climate was milder and wetter and bones of extinct animals found in the area confirm the drastic modifications Gobustan has undergone.[21] Sagona (2018) suggests that a site like this "with its concentration of petroglyphs, revisited a multitude of times over the millennia, must have had social and emotional meanings that were deeply embedded in its features and in the psyche of the people," an aspect that highlights "the sense of place and its implications for identity and meaning, and ultimately for the wellbeing of its users" (78). While at the outer cultural layer, the depiction of weapons and tools (e.g., a type of hoe) is explicit, visualizations of artifacts, illustrations of ritual dances and of half-human-half-animal beings provide insights about other crucial aspects of survival (e.g., at a spiritual level). Humans with zoomorphic features might be a reference to members of the community with specific functions or endowed with special powers or skills, such as shamans and healers. After all, shamanism is a theme identified in visual *art* from prehistoric to modern-day times.[22] Perhaps the petroglyphs did not indeed seek to mediate, express, or describe the lives of those hunters who drew them, but rather to serve as catalyzers for particular rituals or performative actions. One thing is for sure, the omission of unimportant details indicates intentionality. Images are laboriously pecked on a boulder for a reason or to serve a purpose. One might assume that the final result must somehow succeed in expressing what the makers intend to encapsulate and inscribe pictographically. The petroglyph of a group of pregnant women, for example, focuses on a cluster of individuals sharing as commonality their state of gestation. The drawing can be interpreted as the portrayal of a ceremony, of a moment of camaraderie and companionship, or perhaps of a gathering of women from different places, coming together to visit the local midwife. These are, of course, only speculations and attempts to make sense of the raison d'être behind its creation. The mediation mechanisms of prehistoric images remain a mystery, although they retain their pertinence.

When briefly discussing the Upper Paleolithic anatomical drawing of an elephant showing the accurate position of the heart, found in Cueva del Pindal (Oviedo, Spain), Archer (1989) suggests that it serves a didactic purpose. It is probably there for the "benefit of the artist's fellow hunters" (51). Knowing the exact position of the heart mattered to them. Applying a similar pedagogical lens to the Gobustan petroglyphs for modern-day audiences, they can be seen as evidence of ecological, climatic, and cultural change. Less wet conditions presumably imply important modifications in not only the fauna but also vegetation found in the area. From this standpoint, it is possible to conclude that the use of plants observed throughout the many stages of the petroglyph regeneration would have undergone important changes as well. Today, different from the images, long boats, at least in the vicinity of the site, are rare and aurochs (*Bos primigenius*) do not roam around any longer.[23] The figures of animals were important in terms of health, as they presumably tended to represent or allude to a state of well-being.[24]

A connection between the first example and the second one (figure 0.3), Cholpon-Ata petroglyph site (Kyrgyzstan) is the depiction of animals as a theme in petroglyphs. While across the Caucasus, for instance, there seems

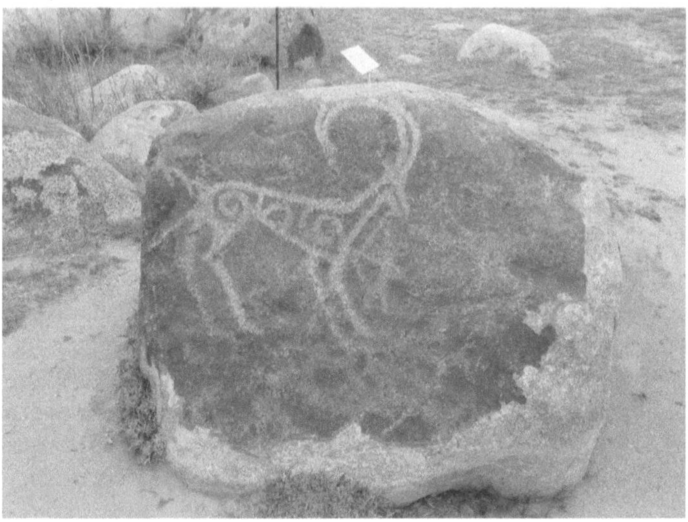

Figure 0.3 One of the Petroglyphs Depicting Animals found in Cholpon-Ata, Kyrgyzstan. *Source*: Photo taken by author during a visit to the Cholpon-Ata petroglyph site, colloquially known as Stone Garden, in 2016.

to have been a cult surrounding the ibex, aurochs had a special place in Central Asian cosmologies as markers of abundance and fertility.[25] As in the case of Gobustan, in Cholpon-Ata, even if these petroglyphs are apparently visually accessible to us today, many of the mysteries inscribed in the actual creation of these images might never be resolved. Their original role within the culture(s) to which they belong are undecipherable to us (with accuracy), precisely because they express a relation that escapes those for whom the petroglyphs are not intended, either as viewers, users, witnesses, worshippers, co-creators, or co-participants. The variety of media, formats, genres, and approaches to the visualization of the nature-health dyad in cultural representations is broad. To the boulders, rocks and stones discussed earlier, one might add bamboo, silk, and metal, used by Egyptians, Babylonians, Chinese, and Indians, as materials used to illustratively register these civilizations' knowledge about the anatomy, care, and cure of the human body.[26]

At the same time, many of the visual representations of health can be considered as implicit recorded passages of interspecies interaction (co-evolutions), even if they champion an anthropocentric standpoint. Animals are a common theme found in pictorial attempts to encapsulate or symbolically represent human life (and the supernatural). Deducing from the abundance of visual representations portraying animals, it is easy to realize that they occupy a special place in epistemic systems dominated by intergenerational traditional knowledge, as much as in those informed by scientific inquiry.[27] As observed by Woods et al. (2018), understanding the part of animals in the evolution of medicine is "more than simply add animals to existing medical historical narratives" as they "also have the potential to reconfigure understandings of what medicine was, and therefore what medical history might become" (245). Tracing interspecies interaction throughout the centuries involves understanding the role of nonhuman beings as historical figures in their own right.[28] Pictorial renderings of hunting, domestication, and husbandry inherently highlight the function of animals within the repertoire of survival strategies and innovations devised by human societies.[29] Paradoxically, creating and maintaining ecosystems in which human life relies heavily on animals (e.g., through intensive factory farming), on a long term, poses nevertheless one of the biggest threats to life on Earth.[30] Moreover, by the time this book is being drafted, a pandemic such as the one prompted by COVID-19 reminds us of the implications of human-animal interaction (co-evolutions) from a health perspective.[31] Coronavirus is a recent example, but risk of zoonotic infections and transmission of diseases is not new in the horizon. Neither are concerns about the ecological implications of changes in land use, exploitation of wildlife, predatory behaviors, and deforestation.

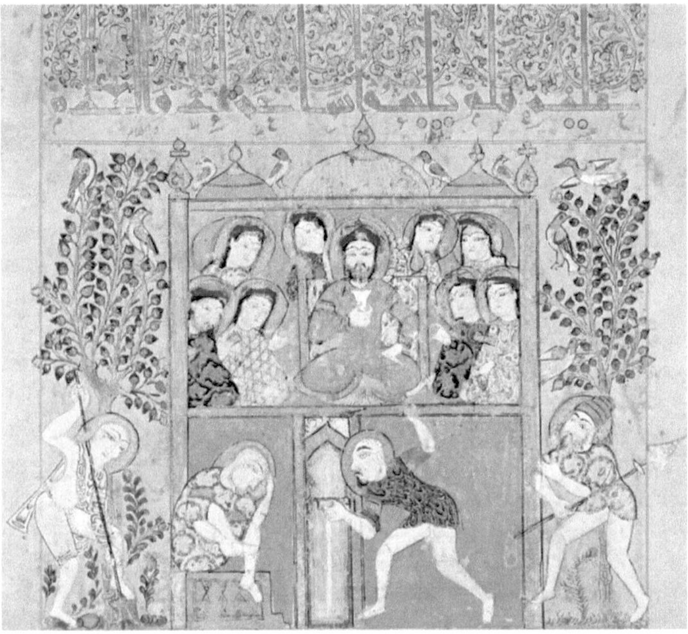

Figure 0.4 Enslaved Prisoner Bitten by a Snake at the Prince's Palace. *Kitāb al-Diryāq* (كتاب الدرياق .)/ *Book of Antidotes* (1198–1199). *Source*: The Yorck Project (2002), Directmedia.

Throughout the centuries, images have served as outlets to express social attitudes toward animals, anxieties about their possible dangers, and appreciation of their applicability as materia medica or as health-enhancing precursors. As the next example illustrates (figure 0.4), the interspecies coexistence as a visual theme features in different ways. In this illustration, originally published in *Kitāb al-Diryāq* (كتاب الدرياق.)/*Book of Antidotes* (1198–1199), the snake might not seem prominent, but it is fundamental to interpret the image.

The painting shows a slave in the lower section recovering from an overdoses of opium by virtue of a snake's bite, which acts as the antidote agent for the reduced state of consciousness caused by the stupefacient. In the upper section of the composition, a prince is unmindful of the situation taking place in the basement of his palace. A workman performs the role of witness to the effect of the reptile's bite in reanimating an intoxicated person. The painting can be interpreted from various perspectives, but above all, it is the illustration of an antidote being used as the materialization of expertise about substances. About the differences in approaches between two copies of the same manuscript, Pancaroğlu (2001) asserts that the *Kitāb al-Diryāq* preserved in Paris

> "is a true milestone not just because it stands at the beginning of a long tradition of illustrated manuscripts but especially because it is one of the most complete testaments to the intellectually conceived and popularly disseminated visual humanism of the late Seljuq period" (170).

In her analysis of the book, Pancaroğlu warns us about the tendency of dismissing the didactic functionality of health-related sceneries in images.[32] Nonetheless because illustrations, such as this one, exemplify the role of visual surfaces in "socializing medicine" (Pancaroğlu, 2001). An aspect of visual representations, I argue, is as present and relevant in a twelfth-century manuscript, as in a modern-day infographic (see chapter 3).

The illustration from the *Book of Antidotes* touches, even if that is a secondary theme, also on the topic of agency and care. One might argue that the inclusion of the snake is in itself an instrument to revive the intoxicated slave, as much as proof of a bystander's involvement in providing some type of medical assistance. Care and healing as themes are major subjects in art, nonetheless because of the overtly religious connection made between the notions of disease, mercy, sin, punishment, miracle, and divine intervention. In Western art, attending the sick has, among others, inspired Bonaventura Berlinghieri (*Miracle of Saint Francis Healing Bartholomew of Narni*, ca. 1235), Fra Angelico (*Healing of the Deacon Justinian*, c. 1440), Jan Sanders van Hemessen (*Tobias Restores His Father's Sight*, 1555), Palma il Giovane (*Christ Healing the Paralytic at Bethesda*, 1592), Antonio Bellis (*Saint Sebastian Tended by Saint Irene*, 1640–1645), Pierre Subleyras Hubert (*San Camillo de Lellis Saves the Sick in the Hospital of the Holy Spirit*, 1746), Luigi Nono (*Convalescence*, 1889), Dean Cornwell (*Conquerors of Yellow Fever*, c. 1939), and evocatively René Magritte (*The Healer*, 1962). Besides the provision of care, an underlying idea easily extracted from the *Book of Antidotes* painting is the centrality of traditional knowledge. Bearing in mind the social position and status of the workers in the basement, graphically allocated by the artist at the lowest level of the palace, they are not presumed to have been scholars, doctors, or members of an intellectual circle. The image in the *Kitāb al-Diryāq* implies that knowing how to use a snake as a remedy against intoxication was (or should have been) part of the vernacular medicinal repertoire of the community. Or else, as Pancaroğlu observes that the illustration had the goal or capacity to disseminate information, didactically instructing viewers or alerting them about what to do in such a situation (i.e., opium overconsumption episode).

Health relies on knowledge and vice versa. The need to understand, respond, and react to medical concerns remains a cornerstone in most epistemic systems. As the fourth example shows, the characterization of medicine includes the creation of images intended to serve a didactic and informative

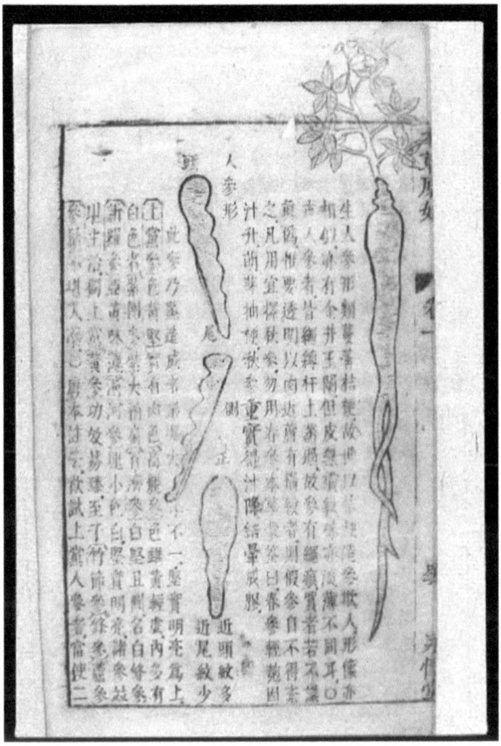

Figure 0.5 本草原始 (*Origins of Materia Medica*), C17: Plant Drugs, Ginseng (genus: *Panax*) (人蔘). *Source*: Wellcome Collection. Public Domain Mark.

purpose. Figure 0.5 is an illustration and description of ginseng's medicinal properties from 本草原始 (*Origins of Materia Medica*), written by Li Zhongli (printed in 1596), "The first illustrated handbook containing observational drawings of medicinal substances (in their raw state) to be published in China."[33] Although specifically, this image comes from the edition published in 1638. The context is important. As Schemmel (2020) observes, knowledge accrued during the Ming (明) dynasty survived after its eventual replacement by the "Qing 清 dynasty, a Manchurian foreign rule" (4). This epistemic continuity included, for instance, the preservation of *Origins of Materia Medica.* On this account, the manuscript contains images that are testament to the role of visual production as a form of knowledge preservation and dissemination.

Images, such as this page about ginseng,[34] along with artifacts and practices have the capacity to encapsulate knowledge, and while they move along, they occupy spaces that denote the tangibility or intangibility of elements or parts, either minimal or substantial, of the epistemic systems where they emerge. Knowledge about ginseng eventually reached other parts of the world.

The mobilization of information about ginseng (genus: *Panax*) (人蔘), and its properties from Asia to Europe, along with the transportation of the actual species, remains evidence of the global circumvolution of knowledge.[35] The introduction of ginseng in the European materia medica repertoire was received with anticipation, generating reactions from scholars, and intensifying its eventual dissemination through various channels.[36] In France, for instance, there were localized, but vociferous debates about its efficacy. While it was commercialized as a panacea imported from the Far East, it did not seem to convince all members of the scientific community.[37] During the nineteenth century, the presence of ginseng as a theme in French print media prompted a sense of curiosity and speculation.[38] Advertisement used to promote "miraculous" formulas, such as ginseng wine, underlined the Oriental and ancient origin of the plant.

One of the rhetoric tools to contextualize ginseng-based products was to imply a connection between distant geographies and the embodiment of traditional wisdom. The allure of little-known corners of the globe, such as Tartary, served to channelize, or perhaps, to thwart any doubt about its medicinal properties.[39] Visually, Chinese characters in packages, labels, leaflets, and promotional material fulfilled an ornamental purpose. Graphically, the distinctiveness of a different writing system marked and guaranteed the Oriental origin of the product being sold. As Mr. Sarniguet, the distributor of the 20-franc-ginseng-wine bottles explains in 1851, "du moment que ces bouteilles sont accompagnées d'une notice imprimée en langue chinoise, il est évident que l'usage de ce vin doit vous rendre centeinaire" (as long as these bottles are accompanied by a notice printed in the Chinese language, it is obvious that the use of this wine must make you a centenarian).[40] According to this, the function of the characters was indexical, ornamental, and epistemic. The inclusion of Chinese revolved around its "pictograph-ness," a term I use in the book to refer to the qualities of visual surfaces to merge texts and images as pictorial strategies.

Today, even if partially, ginseng is epistemically present in the life of those involved in its dissemination, commercialization, exploitation, reutilization, and applicability. It is a remedy, a commodity, and an industry estimated to have mobilized over USD 19.5 million in 2018.[41] Even if research on the medical properties of ginseng is inconclusive, its visual and virtual (i.e., social media) presence reflects its wide popularity as a herbal remedy across the world.[42] The visibility of assumptions about ginseng is engendered in illustrations embedded in communicational strategies, or as contextualizing substratum for the mobilization of end-products, mostly derived from commercial endeavors. An example thereof is the line of coconut-oil- and ginseng-enhanced gum-strengthening dental products launched by Colgate®

in 2020 in Latin America and Spain. The inclusion of *jenjibre* (ginseng) as an antibacterial agent is there to tap into preconceived ideas about its efficacy.[43] To which degree can ginseng contribute to the care of sensitive gums can hardly be determined from the images and texts of the promotional ads. Yet, the materiality of the packages containing the toothpaste, their visual surfaces, labels, and outer packaging are nevertheless physical evidence of an epistemic transfer—of some sort—taking place centuries ago. Recognizing that information transfers occur in incomplete, fragmented, misinterpreted, partial, or paradoxical ways raises questions on *how* knowledge is interpreted, *when*, and *whose* traditional knowledge is valued.

Other Knowledge(s) and Science(s)

While the previous four examples focus on images that presumably portray characterizations of the nature-knowledge-health triad from an insider's perspective, the next two revolve around representations of epistemic systems alien to the intended audience. The composition of the images suggests that by depicting elements of *other knowledges and sciences*, their creators provide cues about their own epistemologies. These are visual surfaces, I argue, that tacitly expose how bioclusivity canons precede, inform, and embed attitudes about other forms of knowing or understanding the world. The kind of encounters these images create bring to mind observations made by Schaffer (2009), on the initial British responses to the construction of observatories in Jaipur (Northern India) in the eighteenth century. Confronted with perplexing astronomical advances, it seemed more logical to the explorers to credit an ancient civilization for its scientific sophistication than to assume that epistemic systems could emerge, evolve, and flourish in parallel. Denying the coevalness of scientific progress seemed easier than recognizing the magnitude of non-European contemporary achievements.[44] The kind of dismissal I identify in some of the images discussed throughout the book, and in which the main focus lies on "distant" and "exotic" medicinal traditions. It is indeed not only a matter of course characteristic of the eighteenth century. This is an approcah Konadu (2008) underlines in his discussion of foreign academics doing fieldwork in Africa. Kwasi observes that non-African anthropologists fail to describe and understand Akan medicine, precisely because they misinterpret elements that seem foreign to them. Konadu's point does not revolve around images, but it does touch upon the general picture sketched by researchers working in context that is not their own. He is critical about "the failure to locate African perspectives on therapeutic matters" in scholarly enterprises designed to carry out observations "*in* the field," but without echoing the context "*of* the field (i.e., Africa)" (46). Konadu asserts that

> in reducing African medicinal systems to "witchcraft," global readers and Africans consume such anthropological or colonial renderings of those systems and, invariably, fail to appreciate the layers of indigenous (medicinal) knowledge possessed by various members of a community and the ideational basis of the systems' approach and therapy. (54)

A lens that can be easily identified throughout the images and artifacts discussed in this book where the focus is to (re)present an epistemic system from an outsider's point of view. A case in point is illustrated in the next example (figure 0.6).

It is one of the wood engraving drawings that accompanies the discussion about cupping among the Angolese in John George Wood's *The Natural History of Man: Africa* (1868).[45] Based on David Livingstone's accounts,[46] Wood contextualizes the illustration by observing that

> some parts of Angola are low, marshy, and fever-breeding, and even the natives feel the effects of the damp, hot, malarious climate. Of medicine, however, they have but little idea, their two principal remedies being cupping and charms. The former is a remedy which is singularly popular, and is conducted in much the same way throughout the whole Africa south of the equator. (Wood, 1868, 423)

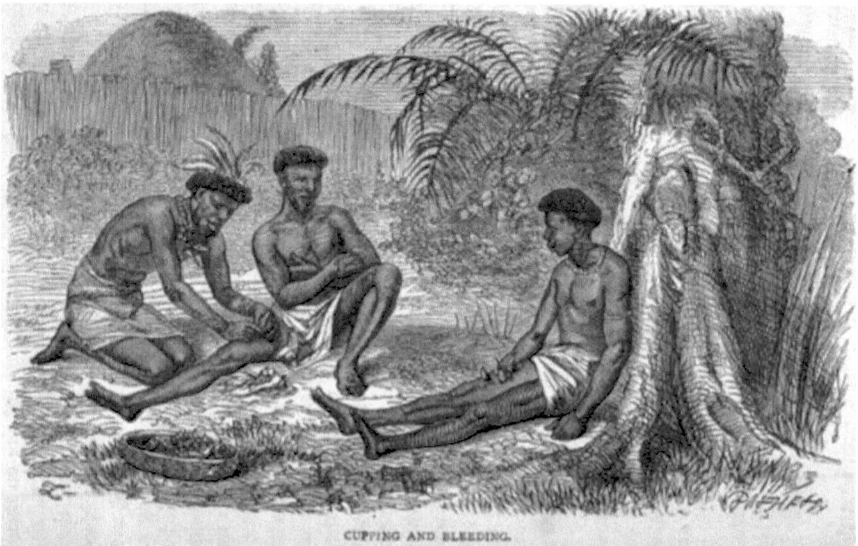

Figure 0.6 An African Medicine Man Cupping and Bleeding Two Patients. Wood engraving (unspecified date) by Dalziel after J. Leech (1817–1864). *Source*: Wellcome Collection. Public Domain Mark.

The book subtitle, *Being an Account of the Manners and Customs of the Uncivilized Races of Men*, certainly provides an idea of the author's approach and of the context in which it was written and published. The author, Reverend Wood (1827–1889), was a clergyman and writer, considered to have made contributions to the popularization of science in Victorian England.[47] Although there are discrepancies on how to measure the outreach and popularity of his publications, some of Reverend Wood's books gained undoubtedly notoriety within certain social circles.[48]

The image is commonly attributed to John Leech (1817–1864), a renown caricaturist of the Victorian Era. Nevertheless, records compiled by the Dalziel brothers, the wood engravers in charge of producing the book, indicate that Johann Baptist Zwecker (1814–1876) was the one commissioned to make the illustrations. A "Z" in the corner convinces me even more to suggest that the wood engraving is actually authored by Zwecker, as part of the assignment requested by Routledge. Based on Dalziel's records, it is most likely that the drawing dates from 1861 to 1863. The authorship of the illustration argumentatively does not seem to matter to the discussion advanced by Wood about the backwardness of Angolese medicinal practices in the nineteenth century. It is nevertheless important to mention that cupping as a therapeutic technique has been part of the medicinal repertoire of many civilizations (e.g., Egyptians, Chinese, and Greeks) for hundreds of years.[49] Records show that by the time Wood's book was published, bleeding was still practiced in Europe.[50] In fact, Leech, the presumed author of the drawing, was one of many patients who received cupping sessions as part of a therapy against severe inflammatory attacks during his childhood.[51] The Dalziel brothers assert that every illustration was made according to the instructions provided by the author. If Reverend Wood indeed instructed the illustrator on how and what to depict to portray the notions of "Cupping and bleeding," the caption assigned to the image in the book (page 423), Leech—if he was the illustrator—had probably replied that he knew what cupping actually entailed. It was not only an *Angolese remedy.*

Reverend Wood's book was nonetheless not the first work devoted to the human diversity that included passages and images on the distinctiveness and questionability of traditional medicinal knowledge. Actually, Wood's *The Natural History of Man: Africa* was preceded by celebrated ethnologist and anthropologist James Cowles Prichard's *The Natural History of Man*, published more than two decades earlier.[52] In his influential work, and building on David Cranz's *Historie von Grönland* (1765),[53] Prichard notes:

> The natives of Greenland were strongly imbued with the notions so prevalent among mankind in different regions, that there must be a particular class of men fitted to mediate between the people and the supernatural powers. These persons

> were termed *angekoks*, that is, sorcerers and diviners. Many families living together, according to Crantz, keep an *angekok* as their counsellor on particular occasions; and if they cannot get one, they are despised and pitied as miserable wretches. In order to become an *angekok*, it is necessary to abandon for a long time the intercourse of men, to macerate the body by long fasting, and by strenous intensity of thought, and, like the Indian sannyasis performing *poojah*, to distract the mind almost into madness. When a *torngak*, or familiar spirit, is obtained by these efforts, the individual becomes an angekok, and thenceforward is possessed of the powers of sorcerers and magicians. On all occasions of distress or sickness the *angekoks* are applied to for relief. It is believed that they can take diseases off or lay them on; that they can call blessings down or chase spectres away. If they have to do with a sick patient, they must mutter something over him, and blow upon him to cure him; or they must fetch and implant a healthy soul in him, or perhaps only predict if he will recover or die. By other enchantments, they discover if an absent man is living or dead. They cite the soul of a man to appear before them; and if they wound such a soul with a spear, the man must die a lingering death. The witches of Greenland are exactly parallel to the witches of England, according to the belief of our ancestors. (Prichard, 1843, 506)

Through comparisons and descriptions, Prichard's main argument is that an inquiry into the inward nature of all races suffices to demonstrate the monogenic origin of humankind.[54] *The Natural History of Man* can of course only be read in the backdrop in which it was drafted without forgetting that this work would eventually influence "many future core texts on topics relating to scientific race studies and human evolution."[55] Methods have evolved as well as interpretations of how others understand their own health landscapes, the role of nature in their procurement of well-being and the capacity of visual expression to register their worldviews. In hindsight, perhaps, neither Wood nor Prichard could fully understand the cultures they sought to describe, and their informants, Livingstone and Cranz, could not have managed to convey or transmit an insider's point of view either. In the context of (forced or not) global exchanges and colonization, reactions, adoption of, and authoritativeness toward therapeutic methods denote that traditional knowledge, I argue, is culturally relatable, epistemologically decipherable, and ontologically interpretable. From this angle, I underline, Cranz, Prichard, Livingstone, or Wood could not have possibly interpreted fully how Angolese or Greenlanders experienced the role of nature and culture in their medicinal repertoires. More importantly, the encompassing epistemic regimes through which they filtered their observations (or interpretations of others' observations) presumably prevented them from understanding the depth and embeddedness of Angolese and Greenlandic traditional knowledge. This does not mean that highlighting the sense of difference or framing as inferior or strange

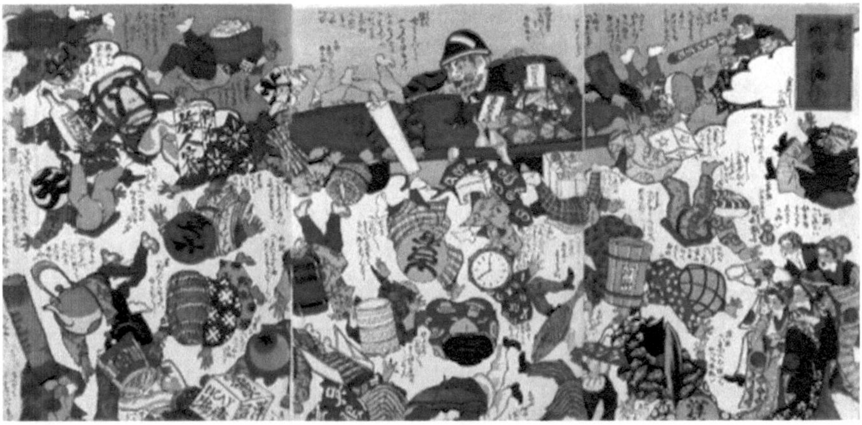

Figure 0.7 A Westerner Capsizing a Boat Out of Which Tumble Commodities of Various Sorts. *Source*: Color woodcut by Baiju Kunitoshi, 1883 [Utagawa Kunitoshi (1847–1899) 歌川国利 (歌川邦年)]. Wellcome Collection. Public Domain Mark.

is a canon only identified in Western visual culture or print media. I do not suggest by any means that exotification or self-exotification are necessarily linked to Eurocentric ideologies (see chapter 3). The sixth and last example is intended to make precisely that point.

Figure 0.7 symbolically displays the event of a Westerner whose boat has capsized and out of which commodities of all sorts twist and tumble into Japanese waters. When Utagawa Kunitoshi (歌川国利) (1847–1899) created this woodblock triptych in 1883, he was probably fully aware that his country was undergoing a process of significant changes. Even from his position as a "second-rate" artist,[56] working with a printmaking technique in decline, through iconic references, Utagawa Kunitoshi skillfully encapsulates a moment in the Meiji Era (明治). Objects such as the clock, kettle, and crate of foreign-manufactured goods floating in the water, as well as the telescope held by one of the Westerners witnessing the scene intuitively, make a passing allusion to technology. In specific, a type of technology that was transforming Japan in unprecedented ways—originally conceived and developed abroad. In stark contrast, a bale of rice, a cask of sake, and pieces of radish make reference to nature and local customs. A straw mat and a kimono cloth evoke ideas about tradition. All three themes mirror the climate of change brought about by industrialization and socioeconomic reforms, intrinsically linked to the interaction between Japan and the West in the nineteenth century.

This woodblock triptych can be considered as an artwork by a Meiji print artist, and at the same time, it can also be regarded as a visual testimony by Yamamura Kiyosuke, Utagawa Kunitoshi's real name.[57] The image offers a reflection of the state of affairs and how objects are interwoven with exchanges at a global scale, knowledge production, and attitudes. It focuses on the centrality of commodities, such as radish (*Raphanus raphanistrum*, subsp. *Sativus*) and rice (*Oryza sativa*), in interaction with artifacts derived from advances in European science and technology. The bale of rice is meaningful as its price dropped by half in the Tokyo market in the context of the Matsukata deflation (1881–1885),[58] an economic crisis that most certainly affected Utagawa Kunitoshi in many ways. The print is a visual reminder of the significance of artifacts as epistemic tokens, either agricultural (e.g., rice), artisanal (e.g., kimono), or technical (e.g., clock), and also as embodiments of foreign knowledge, approaches, and innovations. The concept of modernity is linked to the circulation and material presence of objects. After all, this is the tale of a Westerner whose plan to transport various types of Japanese and non-Japanese commodities fails. In his print, Utagawa Kunitoshi offers a critique of artifacts as markers of modernity and as epistemic repositories, reminding us of the centrality of material artifacts in the restructuration of epistemic systems. At the same time, the triptych prompts a reflection on how visual surfaces play a role in the mediation and dissemination of knowledge, nonetheless through the inclusion of relatively trivial objects.

As I hope to show in the subsequent chapters, references to nature and health found in, for instance, children's toys, a social media post, a stamp, or a souvenir magnet contain despite their mundaneness traces of the epistemic canons of their makers. Understanding health and nature as a theme in present-day mediascapes depends on realizing that its visual presence is, to a large extent, coupled with the images and objects that inform these representations and with the knowledge behind their production.

Mediation of Knowledge, Science, and Health

A utopic state of immutable perfect health has not been reached by any civilization yet, which explains how deployment of knowledge and developments of methods to counteract illness have followed humanity from the beginning of times. Caring for and curing the body matters because it conditions any other faculty or capability. Any attempt to express our human condition visually is preceded by attending to our bodily needs first and, to a certain extent, our sense of well-being. The contemporary use of media to purvey ideas and present novelties to cure medical conditions aligns with a tradition of documenting, preserving, and sharing knowledge.[59] Dissemination/appropriation of information about the properties of cinchona in the sixteenth century (genus *Cinchona*), for example, is evidence of the potentiality of local ethnobotanical practices to treat health problems at a global scale—mirroring eventually, nevertheless, also the dark side of environmental decimation and depletion of resources. The case of cinchona, as the basic ingredient of antimalarials, prompts a reflection about the multifaceted reality of epistemic transfers.[60] If colonization of new territories means the colonization of knowledge as Boumediene (2018) has shown, the contextualization of current bioprospecting projects raises many questions in terms of power relations, economic disparities, and neocolonialism.[61] A history that is inscribed in the long tradition of producing knowledge, conditioned by hierarchies superimposed on peripheral epistemic systems. As Schiebinger (2017) shows, in the case of eighteenth-century transatlantic networks of cures, subjects for experimentation and commodities.[62] All forms of knowledge evolve and so does their applicability within the contexts in which they are produced. As Margócsy (2014) observes in his detailed study of the commodification of images in the Dutch Golden Age, and yet pertinent still today, "Scientific consensus is overturned eventually, as knowledge accumulates across the centuries, but philosophical arguments, and the commercial context that sets them in motion, recur again and again" (216).

The commercial is indeed prominent. The foremost contact points between societies and manifestations of scientific advances are items and phenomena we encounter every day. As much as a photo of a black hole taken in space thousands of miles away or the microscopic image of an atom's shadow impacts, impresses, and rewrites history. It is the commodifiable, abstract, and yet tangible knowledge behind objects, such as a mobile phone, or baby infant formula, that seems to revolutionize our existence through their mundane invasion of the spaces we inhabit. As Rentetzi's *epistemology of the familar* (2020, 38) so compellingly alerts us about. The onus lies in recognizing that this knowledge is inherently embedded in social, economic, and political systems. The possibility of using a device that enables us to communicate with others or of accessing a powder that mimics human milk are practices derived from epistemic processes, materialized in artifacts through the creation of networks of production and distribution. While (pure/fundamental/basic) science aims at understanding, theorizing, and formulating explanations and predictions related to the physical world, applied science aims at solving nontheoretical issues or at operationalizing the use of accrued knowledge in one way or another. Even if science and applied science seem to answer different questions, they both depend on economic constraints to exist and hereby on the recognition of their value for the advancement of humanity. The economics of both types of science is crucial to understand their dynamics with the societies they serve and their presumed absence in societies where the notion of knowledge is understood differently. A law of physics, until it is falsified, overruled by a new paradigm, or a more refined explanation, is bound to retain its dominancy. The "tradition-shattering" episodes complement scientific "tradition-bound" activities in Kuhn's terms (1962, 6).

At a structural level, the inception of artifacts and epistemic practices, such as those derived from scientific discoveries, can potentially reconfigure societies. The normalization of new additions in the compendium of material and immaterial epistemic repertoires denotes the human tendency to learn, or unlearn, depending on how one looks at it. It is undeniable that the mobilization of knowledge and its objects has changed the face of the Earth. In the process, it has had an impact on the intimate relation societies have with their environments and their understandings of themselves within their dwellings. The ability to organize, restructure, design, and plan spaces lies at the core of economic, political, and social projects that have changed the world, in many ways, perhaps for the worse. Current economic models have side effects that, at times, seem diametrically opposite to the conservation and preservation of natural habitats. Pollution, extractivism, excessive use of unrenewable sources of energy, deforestation, and uncontrolled use of CO_2-producing devices (from motorbikes to planes) has left us with an ecological crisis of unsurmountable scale—a crisis that is bound to affect the health and chances of survival of millions. Mass production/consumption of resources and objects, their distribution across the globe, and their eventual disposal have disbalanced the equilibrium of the entire planet in unprecedented ways.

Objects have emerged as extensions and derivatives of the human beings that use them. They serve a purpose known to their masters. The creation of a wooden statue and the preparation of a meal resemble each other in the sense that both stem from the knowledge needed to maneuver cuttings from a tree and the selection and mixture of raw ingredients. The fabrication of a measurement equipment, a syringe, or an anesthesia machine is no different. Knowledge lies behind their manufacturing and a need (or accident) lies behind their conception, development, and circulation. All along, a society retains a view about those tools, objects, and inventions. They belong to one category or other within the imaginary, memory, and tradition of each community. The circulation of objects interculturally is one of the social practices that has shaped our existence since the beginning of times. Exchanges of artifacts involve sharing experiences and knowledge engrained in their production and adoption. Eventually, they materialize in externalizations and visual characterizations.

With the onset of new technologies, the availability of instruments that facilitate the creation of visual cultural artifacts has reconfigured canons and modes of diffusion of knowledge. In the context of health-enhancing and health-restoring treatments and therapies, objects with medicinal properties, or presented as such, move across communicational networks with a speed never seen before.[63] Swiftness in the production of visuals has amplified the availability of information on the various approaches to health that societies around the world distinctively deploy, recognize, or trust. A notoriously augmented flow of content does not mean every image, infographic, or vlog accurately mirrors how target audiences understand the care and cure of the body.[64] Neither does it imply that the information conveyed, for instance, in informally (homemade) constructed videos follows standards of veracity, accuracy, or scientific rigor, most commonly observed by scientists, health professionals, legal institutions, and scholars.[65] Nevertheless, the availability and popularity of videos about traditional knowledge(s) suggest that audiences are interested in exploring epistemic practices that might not necessarily align with conventional research-based biomedicine.

Today more than ever, moving, still images and mundane artifacts operate as catalyzers for the diffusion of information about health. Progressively, it has become a difficult task, at times, to distinguish between a genuine informative video clip and an advanced form of indirect advertisement. Economic interests play a role in the promotion of products commercialized for their effectivity in the treatment of mild and serious conditions. Rules vary considerably between countries, but from a legal perspective, many products remain on a gray area in terms of regulations and protection of potential consumers.[66] Audiences are ultimate the ones in charge of making decisions, but there is certainly a degree of influence exerted by visual media. Media outlets are saturated with images of herbal medicines, medicinal oils, plant-based substances, homemade remedies, nutritional supplements, and elixirs of all sorts.[67]

A notoriously problematic aspect of widespread (mis)information facilitated by images is that it prompts a sense of skepticism that risk eclipsing valuable exchanges and additions of knowledge between small communities and large societies at a micro- and macro-level. Despite extremely difficult circumstances and challenging line of events, myriad forms of traditional bodies of knowledge remain an integral part of the spectrum of dependencies between members of a community and elements of the natural world (bioclusivity). Either orally, and in less degree, through written records, expertise on the use of natural resources for medicinal and therapeutic purposes has been partially preserved. In the context of the current environmental and sanitary crises, peripheral bodies of knowledge are gaining recognition, or at least visibility, among other venues through cultural artifacts discussed in this book. As the next chapters show, the realm of the visual reflects the complex relation societies have with nature as an agent, instrument, ally, catalyzer, potentiator, and source of health. As I show, elements from the natural world, varying from society to society, can be simultaneously placed in the categories of precursors of health and of abstractions of nature, with only those knowledgeable in a particular ontological order being aware of this shifting duality. A common characteristic identified in the corpus is the heterogeneousness in format and content, but the uniformity of mediatization and mediation as pillars in the circulation of ideas about nature as a precursor in the care and cure of the human body.

STRUCTURE OF THE BOOK

The book is divided into three parts, each subdivided into two chapters. The first part, "Images of Nature," considers the ways in which visual culture operates as a vehicle to diffuse, transmit, mediate, and communicate health-related knowledge and imaginaries about the role of nature as a healing precursor. In chapter 1, "Visual Healing," the discussion revolves primarily around a Mexican fiction feature film, a Guatemalan documentary, and a set of interviews with Mayan midwives. The commonality between these mediatic productions is the rendering of practices embedded in Mesoamerican medicinal epistemic systems. The example taken from fiction is included as an entry point for a discussion about the hierarchies of medicinal traditions that underpin present-day health systems. On this account, the three narratives offer a reflection of how cultures adopt elements from their habitats in the creation of strategies to pursuit health or to engage with natural events, such as births.

Along a similar line, chapter 2, "Animated Epistemologies," explores the pictoriality of objects designed to have a didactic or semiotic role. On the one hand, by focusing on animated series, toys, and children's books, this chapter emphasizes the epistemic role of educational, instructive, and ludic material in the mediation of information about health and nature. A French animated series, a Danish line of action figurines, and children's visual dictionaries in thirty-five languages from all corners of the globe are the main objects of study. On the other hand, the discussion of medical philately explores the subthemes through which stamps operate as functional, symbolic, and iconic renderings of idiosyncratic self-representativeness. The focus lies on the various health-related topics addressed in stamps, considering that their functional purpose does not undermine the message wrapped in their chromatically appealing composition. The main thesis of the chapter is that the circulation of ideas depends to a large extent on the semiotic-material dimension of objects. Bearing in mind that acquisition of knowledge at an intergenerational and intercultural level occurs through mediated externalizations, the study cases elucidate in which ways ludic visualizations enact the health-nature dyad.

The second part of the book, "Shapes of Nature," explores the transmogrification process by which nature becomes consumable, encapsulated in objects defined by their visual and material traits.[68] It focuses on items, such as labels on packages of herbal cosmetics and infographics about superfoods. The illustrative dimension is addressed from a tripartite perspective. First, these images can presumably be treated as interpretations or extractions of (un)acknowledged epistemic systems and knowledge transfers. Second, they can presumably play a role in diffusing pieces of (mis)information that navigate across outlets such as the Internet and public spaces. Third, these visual-material artifacts offer a reflection about the interplay between technology, societies, and the natural world. The set of consumables addressed in both chapters is evidence of the general assumption that objects mediate the operationalization of medicinal practices. While chapter 3, "Barcoded Pharmacopeias," concentrates on the promotion of health-enhancing plant-based and fruit-based supplements, chapter 4, "Gendered Epistemic Artifacts," hones in on natural beauty products. This chapter, in particular, looks at the gendered axes that traverse biosocial practices. The corpus of study in "Barcoded Pharmacopeias" are sites of graphic communication surrounding naturality-inspired items sold in North America and Europe, but containing purportedly herbs, plants, barks, seeds, and fruits collected in Africa, Asia-Pacific region, and Latin America. In "Gendered Epistemic Artifacts," the objects of analysis are Korean and Moroccan cosmetics and the visuality and materiality that undergird their mobilization as consumables and receptacles of assumptions about gender, skincare, and naturality.

In "Sites of Nature," the third part of the book, the main vantage point is the situatedness of health within two physical contexts, a geographical and a mental one. On the one hand, chapter 5, "Topological Panaceas," reviews the connection societies make between health and sites endowed with a sense of naturality.[69] On the other hand, chapter 6, "Sensorial Interfaces," discusses the human mind as a working milieu for psychotropics, specifically naturally found mind-altering precursors rooted in cultural, medical, and social practices with legal implications. In both cases, the discussion about the natural world as a source of inspiration focuses on structure and form. Chapter 5 reviews the history of outdoor bathing and swimming (*sund*) in Iceland as a practice that emerged in response to major biosocial, technological, and idiosyncratic developments throughout the nineteenth and twentieth centuries. *Sund* is analyzed through its pictorial and epistemic-semiotic presence in public outlets. Based on a Canadian documentary, the second section of the chapter explores Okanagan medicinal practices. It considers, in specific, the geographic dimension of health as part of epistemologies in which, for instance, a lake operates as a nucleus for a specific healthscape and indigeneity. Along a similar line of thought, chapter 6 briefly chronicles the history of entheogens used by Indigenous communities in Latin America, eventually synthesized and adopted to other uses in European and North American labs. A history that images have documented through sixteenth-century manuscripts, photographs in magazines, works of art, and digital artwork brochures. The focus lies on the tension between the tradition and stigmatization surrounding psychoactive substances for medical and social order reasons. Similarly, in the second part of the chapter, the discussion revolves around cannabis. The departing point is the way in which visual culture has recorded the legalization, implementations, and changes in attitudes toward the psychoactive precursor in The Netherlands and Uruguay. As this chapter intends to show, the mind is part of the topology of health.

Throughout the book, the focus lies on visual representations as articulations of the miscellany of ideas about naturality and health, while remaining attentive to the fact that images can be understood to betoken and semiotically reveal other processes. They are semiotic projections of *a* type of knowledge but not necessarily of data endorsed by evidence-based research. These visual characterizations are nevertheless epistemic in the sense that they reflect objects and practices found in present-day knowledge systems. In my approach, I align with Schemmel's observation that a global history of knowledge "is not helped by facile dichotomies between 'East' and 'West'."[70] In short, the objects of study are epistemic-semiotic visual surfaces where nature and health intersect.

Furthermore, the images/surfaces discussed in this book confirm the tangibleness of strategies deployed by those pursuing to cure and care for their bodies, unmindful of hierarchized systematic paradigms. From a Western scientific perspective, a number of them mobilize vague claims that are not supported by evidence obtained by applying the dominant current scientific method. A fact that does not eclipse their reception among audiences. There is a thin line between health communication, the spread of fake data, dissemination of misinformation, manipulation of visual outlets for commercial purposes, and promotion of media spaces that question or deter evidence- and research-based biomedicine. This book does not seek to compare, contrast, assess, or scrutinize the articulations of cultural repertoires. It is my hope that the argumentation serves as a dialogue between sites of knowledge dissemination. A discussion and references to scientific publications, embedded in the principles of reproducibility and replicability, are used to gloss, contextualize, and moderate the images discussed in the book. It is difficult to assess levels of scientific rigor, unbiasedness, impartiality, and verifiability in studies carried out within the premises of alternative medicine, undisclosed experiments, misinformation, and purely commercial enterprises. The emphasis lies on images that characterize how each social group's bioclusivity primes its use of nature as a precursor of health.

NOTES

1. Throughout the book, I use Jürgen Renn's (2020) definition of knowledge: "The capacity of an individual agent or of a group to solve problems and mentally anticipate or perform corresponding actions. Knowledge is internally represented by cognitive structures, allowing for the connection of past and current experiences. Knowledge is not just experience encoded in individual mental structures; it also has material and social dimensions, allowing human societies to acquire and encode experiences and thereby to share and transmit them over generations" (427).

2. Levinas (1951) explains ontology as a synonym of the whole human being, in view of the fact that, in his own words, "scientific work, the affective life, the satisfaction of needs and labor, social life and death—all these moments spell out the comprehension of being, or truth with a rigor which reserves to each a determinate function" (3). This passage is taken from the English translation, Levinas (1996), a translation of "L'Ontologie est-elle fondamentale?," published in *Revue de métaphysique et de morale* in 1951.

3. Smith 2012.

4. Smith, 2012, 47.

5. In specific, they are present in contexts in which qualitative assessment of data relies on its accuracy, limited by the constraints of classifying cross-referentially, avoiding vagueness or open ends.

6. In explaining how ontology could be applicable in the classification of information and informatic systems, Gruber (1993) asserts that the philosophical term is a "systematic account of existence," or in other words, "an explicit specification of a conceptualization" (199). One in which any inter-operationality can only take place if the taxonomies accurately describe the elements of each domain and their entities.

7. Cornet and Abu-Hanna, 2003.

8. Rosse and Mejino, 2003.

9. In these cases, the basis of creating any information system is establishing in which way data are indexed, defined, and entered. Interfaces that include the textualization of visuals and the visualization of texts (Bard, 2003; Cimino and Zhu, 2006; Jayapandian et al., 2014; Lamy, 2016; Alfonse and Gawich, 2020; Pernisch et al., 2021).

10. Full quote: "As for the history of the whole, I distinguish between the history of the whole as such and the history of the location of the whole, according to the modification and for substitution of its parts. The histories relative to the location of the whole and to the modification or substitution of its parts enable us to establish various criteria of identity (material, functional, etc.)" (Poli, 1996, 318).

11. Charmaz (1991), Nordenfelt (1995), Tarlov (1996), Guerrero (2010), and Venkatapuram (2013).

12. Margolis (1976); Goosens (1980) ; Clouser, Culver, and Gert (1981); Agich (1983) ; Fulford (1989) ; Nordenfelt (1995); and Cooper (2005).

13. Jordanova, 1995, 377.

14. See D'Argenio (2022) and Gonzalez Rodriguez (2022).

15. *Jaibaná Bedea* is a short documentary made as a collective project of Krinchia u Numua—Indigenous Communicational Grassroot Movement, Chigorodó (Colombia). The name of the Finnish film *Kanarialinnut* in English is *Canaries.* The Laotian filmmaker's full name is Namthipkesone Bouttasing.

16. As stated earlier, the focus lies upon naturality, defined as the state of being related to nature, realizing that nature varies in meaning and considering that this variation is precisely what underpins the notion of bioclusivity. A distinction should be made between naturality and the notions of naturalness and unnaturalness, rigorously discussed in Siipi (2008).

17. Here I refer to the kind of "reportorial dimension" discussed by Bleichmar and Schwartz (2019) that conveys images a sense of authoritativeness, veracity, and informativeness.

18. Based on Uranium-series dating, the image found in the Leang Bulu' Sipong 4 cave of the limestone karsts of Maros-Pangkep in South Sulawesi is at least 43,900 years ago (43.9 ka) (Brumm et al., 2021).

19. More specifically: High Pleistocene, Early Holocene, Neolithic stage (ca. VII–VI millennia BC), Chalcolithic period (VI–IV millennia BC), Bronze Age (IV–III millennia BC), Iron Age (II–I millennia BC), and Middle Ages and later period (I–XVIII c.c) (Farajova, 2011; Sagona, 2018).

20. Anati (2001).

21. Some of them include onager (*Equus hemionus*), Mediterranean tortoise (*Testudo graeca*), gazelle (*Gazella Subgutturoza*), and boar (*Sus scrofa*) (Farajova, 2011).

22. Wallis (2019).

23. Besides DNA analyses and archeological findings, visual surfaces provide crucial information for the reconstruction of the history of cattle and its role for humanity in deep time. Out of which is possible to deduce that both taurine cattle (*Bos taurus*) and zebu (*Bos indicus*) "descend from the extinct wild ox or aurochs (*Bos primigenius*)" that ranged from Northern tundra areas to India and Atlantic to Pacific coasts (Ajmo Ajmone-Marsan, Garcia and Lenstra, 2010, 148).

24. Gobustan inhabitants probably worshipped the sun and other animals, such as snakes. In both cases, they were revered for their power (Smithsonian, 2014)

25. Tashbayeva (2001).

26. Calkins, Franciosi, and Kolesari (1999); Tsafrir and Ohry (2001).

27. Traditional knowledge recognizes the role of animals and their well-being to maintain balance, understanding the implications of animals' well-being, for instance, not only for agriculture (Beinart and Brown, 2013) but also for human health. The treatment of human disease with animal-derived substances and formulas of products (zootherapy) has been identified in many cultures all over the world (e.g., Albania, Italy, Nepal, and Spain) (Quave et al., 2010). In terms of scientific research, animals have taken up different roles throughout the history of biomedicine, either as subjects of experimentation (Wilkinson, 1992; Larrère, 2002; Guerrini, 2003), presumed sources of disease (Pearce-Duvet, 2006), and components of materia medica precursors (Lev, 2003). Using animals in laboratory settings raise questions about ethics

(Zurlo, Rudacille and Goldberg, 1994; Baumans, 2004; Cuesta Brey and Sánchez Rodríguez, 2007), which to a certain point, resemble debates that question human consumption of animals as forms of environmental and interspecies violence with serious implications for the future of humanity (Gullone, 2017).

28. Cockram and Wells (2017) offer a multidisciplinary discussion on the various types of relationships that have emerged between humans and animals.

29. This does not mean that the approach to the consumption of by-products of animal slaughter or animal farming has not been vociferously debated from a cultural, ethical, and political angle (Singer, 1997; Graham and Tiffin; 2015; Fischer, 2019; Hölker, von Meyer-Höfer and Achim Spiller, 2019; Dickstein, 2021).

30. Some of the consequence of modern-day factory farming include biodiversity loss, degradation, greenhouse gas emissions, deforestation, and increased use of fertilizers and pesticides needed to supply the feed needs of livestock (Kirby, 2010; Gerber et al., 2015).

31. Soens, De Bont, and De Keyzer (2020) observe that "in its zoonotic origins, in its global spread, in its intrusion of our bodies, practices and infrastructures, COVID-19 proves that the modern ambition to control nature—matured from the 17th century onwards through the Scientific Revolution, Enlightenment, industrialisation and the transition to fossil fuel—has reached its limits" (11).

32. One book is housed in the Bibliotheque Nationale (arabe 29640) (Paris) and the other one in Nationalbibliothek (A.F. 10) (Vienna).

33. Zheng and 鄭金生, 2018, 154.

34. Li Zhongli writes: "Ginseng is found deep in the mountains, in cold, wet places. The young plants are just 3 or 4 cun tall (1 cun [Chinese inch] = c. 3 cm), with five leaves on each shoot. Though they subsequently grow more ramifications, there are only ever five leaves on each of these. The roots are used in medicine. The ones that resemble the human form are the best. It is sweet in sapor, slightly warming in thermostatic character, and non-poisonous. It has the medicinal properties of tonifying the centre and replenishing Qi, generating saliva/bodily fluids and alleviating thirst, recovering from collapse (gu tuo) and calming the mind. It is used to treat over-exertion damage and insufficiency detriment (laoshang xusun), shortness of breath and lack of appetite, fever with spontaneous sweating, insufficiency-overexertion (xulao) with wheezing and panting, distress and restlessness (fanzao) with wasting thirst (xiaoke diabetes), frequent urination and incessant diarrhea, disorders of pregnancy and childbirth, etc" (Wellcome, 2021).

35. Carolus (Carl) Linnaeus followed specific taxonomical protocols to name plants (Müller-Wille, 2006). In the case of ginseng, the Greek meaning of *panax* (Πάναξ) is related to its pressumed "all-healing" properties best articulated by its wide therapeutical and phytopharmaceutical use in traditional Chinese medicine (Skaltsa, 2015).

36. Goldstein (1975), Lee (2016).

37. During the nineteenth century, there is a stark contrast between the sense of speculation and doubt that taint the media attention surrounding the efficacy of ginseng (e.g., *Le Courrier français* and *Le Tintamare*) and advertisement strategies seeking to promote its use (Huart, 1851).

38. See, for instance, *Le Courrier français* (May 1832), *Le Tintamare* (April 1851), and *Le Charivari* (March 1861).

39. Tartary was the umbrella term used to refer to the geographical part of Eurasia known today as Central Asia. Since it was used for over six centuries (thirteenth to nineteenth century), until Western scholars gained more knowledge of the areas comprised between the Caspian Sea, Persia, India, Ural Mountains, and the Pacific Ocean, no ethnic specificity was required to label a person, tradition, or an artifact as Tartarian (de Palafox y Mendoza, 1670; de Guignes, 1756; Clarke, 1848).

40. Huart (1851), 4.

41. Ahuja and Sonal (2018).

42. Lee (2014), Ahuja (2018), Sivasankarapillai (2020), and Alsayari (2021) are among the many studies conducted on the possible medicinal applications of ginseng.

43. This is confirmed by the comments and reviews posted by users on open consumer review platforms. While many of whom praise the ginseng-enhanced dental care products for their effectivity, despite its distinctive taste, others celebrate the use of plant instead of "chemical ingredient."

44. Schaffer (2009) notes that the Eurocentrism of the explorers made it difficult for them not to conclude that technical achievements were part of the legacy of an extinct civilization; one followed by "subsequent degeneration" (89).

45. While the first volume focuses on the African continent, the second volume of Wood's *The Natural History of Man : Being an Account of the Manners and Customs of the Uncivilized Races of Men* discusses Australia, New Zealand, Polynesia, America, Asia, and Ancient Europe (1870).

46. There does not seem to be agreement on how the life and legacy of missionary, explorer, and physician David Livingstone (1813–1873) provided a window into parts of Africa, previously *unknown* to Europeans (Fish and Burost Fish, 2002).

47. Bernard Lightman (2007) notes that although to some, Reverend Wood "was among the preeminent scientific writers of his day" (169), many aspects of his endeavors suggest his attempts to "popularize" science were not entirely successful and that his scholarship might have lacked rigor.

48. In light of several facts, some of the descriptions of success and popularity chronicled by his son, Theodor Wood, in a biography about his father might not be accurate (see Wood, 1890).

49. Prioreschi (1996).

50. Rooney (2013).

51. In his John Leech's biography, Kitton notes that "it is recorded that LEECH in his infancy had a sudden and most severe inflammatory attack, and only the skill of Sir CHARLES MANSFELD CLARK and Dr. JAMES NICHOLLS, humanly speaking, brought him out of it. He used to resist the application of remedies suggested by on one occasion, when he was to be bled by cupping, he baffled the whole domestic force brought against him, until, hearing of his mother's sorrowful disappointment, he jumped up and bade them to do it" (Kitton, 1883, 9).

52. See Augstein (1999) for a discussion on Prichard's contributions to various fields.

53. In *Historie von Grönland enthaltend die Beschreibung des Landes und der Einwohner &c. insbesondere die Geschichte der dortigen Mission der Evangelischen Brüder zu Neu-Herrnhut und Lichtenfels*, German missionary David Cranz (also spelled Crantz) (1723–1777) traces the history of Herrnhuter Büdergemeinde (Moravian Brethren) since their first attempts to evangelize Greenlanders in 1733. The book appeared three years after Cranz returned from Greenland, after spending one year among the Inuits. His interaction with the locals informs many of the descriptions found in *Historie von Grönland* about their epistemologies, traditional knowledge, customs, and worldviews.

54. This is in line with the main conclusion Prichard reaches and defends in *Researches into the Physical History of Mankind* (1813) considered as Prichard's most influential book.

55. Sera-Shriar (2015), 20.

56. Shigeru (2005), 262.

57. Laurance (1976) and Newland et. al (2005).

58. Ericson (2014).

59. Bonah and Laukötter (2020) note that mediatization matters in a time when the channelization of "word-based health politics" has "proven essential for the enactment of beliefs about health and body practices in the communication societies of the 20th century" (14).

60. For the long history of cinchona as medicinal plant, commodity, and biocultural artifact across the Atlantic and throughout Europe, as demonstrated by several studies on the subject (Crawford, 2016; Gachelin et al., 2017; Hokkanen, 2017; Gänger, 2020; Semedo et al., 2021). Cinchona circulated in other colonized territories, exemplifying the impact of commercialization routes as sites for dissemination of medicinal epistemic practices, for instance, in India (Deb Roy, 2017; Tamang et al., 2019).

61. In the second decade of the twenty-first century, decolonization theories have repositioned the role of preservation and production of knowledge. On the matter, Radcliffe and Radhuber observe that "the messy, contested and dynamic political geographies of D/decolonization rupture any assumption that decolonizing is universal or homogeneous, and thereby challenges critical political geographies to pay closer attention to the material and epistemic forces of modernity-coloniality" (2020, 10).

62. Since these are epistemic endeavors with social, economic, corporate, and (politically) representational implications, the terms of the conversation have slightly changed, but still exhort us to wonder, what Hayden asks in her paper in 2005: "What *is* the contribution of 'local' knowledge to the process of drug development? How, in turn, does the relationship between ethnobotanical leads and pharmaceutical measures of value bear on the claims and entitlements that prospecting participants might expect in the future?"(187).

63. Blogs, for instance, as channels to disseminate information about health (Joshi, Wangmo, and Amadi, 2017).

64. Channels, approaches, and techniques for health communication are quite diverse, offer different possibilities, but also challenges (Kreps, 2001).

65. An example thereof is the discussion on an "infodemic" of remedies promoted in vlogs prompted by the COVID-19 pandemic (Banerjee and Meena, 2021).

66. Abundance in media production mirror the abundance of over-the-counter remedies and medicines. See Cooper (2013) for a discussion about the abuse of vaguely regulated medicines internationally.

67. It is often not clear how these categories operate and this is reflected in the visual strategies deployed to promote or simply represent, for instance, food supplements. As Siipi (2020) demonstrates, the distinction between food and supplements is mostly characterized by vagueness.

68. I use Nikki Sullivan's (2006) conceptualization of transmogrification as a trope that "might allow us to acknowledge important similarities, overlaps, resonances, and intersections between a range of modified bodies" (561). However, in the book, I specifically apply the term in specific to *bodies of knowledge* and to the mind as a site that can be transmogrified.

69. In the book, the term "topology" is used to refer to geo-cultural spaces, axiomatically marked by established boundaries defined by idiosyncratic codes, ethnic affiliation, epistemologies, and (im)material heritage.

70. Schemmel, 2020, 2.

Part I

IMAGES OF NATURE

Chapter 1

Visual Healing

Images that explore the nexus between the environment, health, and culture and circulate in media contexts have evolved from being visual representations and portrayals of modus vivendi to becoming dialogic and communicative spaces for exchange and dissemination of knowledge. Cinematic depictions of nature-based healing approaches ultimately become reflections of how societies relate to their local environments. Focusing upon a widely screened fiction feature film from the Golden Age of Mexican Cinema, *María Candelaria* (1944), to a recent Guatemalan short-length documentary, *Rujotay k'aslemal/La vida retoñando a través de la salud/Life Sprouting through Health* (2020), and a series of filmed interviews with Mayan midwives disseminated through open platforms, such as YouTube, this chapter delves into the presentation and representation of Indigenous Mesoamerican medicine. The underlying premise is that the evolution of visual depictions about ethnobotanical practices provides cues about the state of flux that distinguishes the interaction between societies and the natural world. Since the operationalization of treatments involves non-biomedicine practices, a discussion about these media works implies considering the plurality of ontologies of care for the human body and the ecosystems and social contexts in which they take place.

REPRESENTATIONS AND KNOWLEDGE(S)

Visual arts remain intrinsically linked not only to the imaginaries of the producing societies but also to the changes in their epistemic practices and systems. As a European invention, cinematic production became an industry built on Western foundations, and although it has reached all corners of the globe, it remains in many ways heavily dictated by European and North American ideologies.[1] Cultural legacies of old systems where Western values were upheld are still widely present in the industry of entertainment and media. In similar ways, films retain their value as documents that attest the primacy given to specific knowledge(s), ecological models, and understandings about the care and cure of the body. The immanent power of cinema rests in its capacity to have an influence on viewers, reconfigure their perception grid, expand their cultural repertoire, remodel their attitudes, contest their preconceptions, and stimulate their imaginary to visualize a different reality. Films appeal to sensitivities and emotions by prompting a dialogue between the imagery and the mind of the spectators. Visual narratives about Indigenous peoples operate inherently as interpretations of not only their epistemologies but also their place within a social hierarchy dictated by political and economic power.[2]

Cultural representation of Indigenous societies has served to render visible the fact that since the colonization of the Americas, pre-Columbian societies have resided socially and epistemically outside areas of direct influence.[3] Conversely, the figure of the New World native has consistently remained as a trope in Eurocentric visual art, partly informed by generalized ideas Europeans had about distant geographies and peoples and partly based on situations explorers experienced firsthand (figure 1.1).[4] Iconic images of headless men, cannibals, savages, and idyllic natural creatures, allegedly found in the Americas, spread rapidly throughout Europe and beyond, soon after Columbus stepped a foot on San Salvador island in 1492. Nostalgic and phantasmagorical ideas about giants, mermaids, and unicorns were quickly entwined with the natives living in the region. Purportedly, European publishing houses in charge of the edition of drawings, books, and engravings in the sixteenth and seventeenth centuries manipulated the images described or painted by the explorers in order to secure more appealing, awe-inspiring illustrations.[5] A parallel development was the use of images to document the rich biological diversity of flora and fauna of the continent.

Alternatively, the predominant theme in Latin American works of art from the eighteenth century was the various social categorizations found and artificially established in the New World. The birth of new republics instigated not only a sense of belonging but also an inquisitive desire to depict and understand the first civilizations that inhabited the region. When photography and cinema emerged in the nineteenth and early twentieth centuries, young urban nations in Latin America were struggling to define their identity as mestizo societies in a world rapidly being reshaped by technology. Although the first cinematic productions about Central and South America were mainly related to scientific endeavors and ethnographic curiosity (e.g., *Desayuno de indios/Indians' Breakfast*, France-Mexico, 1896), ensuing fictionalized

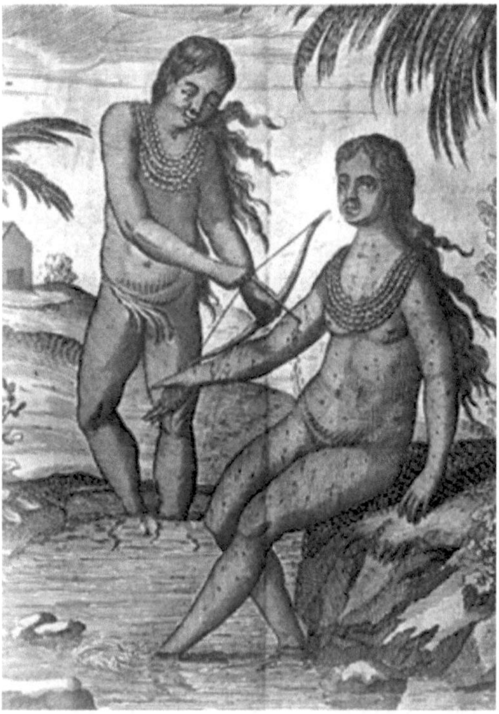

Figure 1.1 Letting Blood by Piercing a Patient's Arm with an Arrow. Indigenous North American. *Source*: Wellcome Collection. Attribution 4.0 International (CC BY 4.0).

productions quickly embraced recycled approaches and tropes that underlined a sense of otherness and difference.[6] Cinema became a tool to optically confirm the striking contrast between rural and urban lifestyles, traditions, and, in some cases, ethnicities (e.g., *Pueblos dormidos/Sleeping Towns*, Argentina, 1947).

In terms of formats, many directors saw documentaries as an appropriate vehicle to mirror the reality of Indigenous communities during the 1960s and 1970s. This was not a novelty, though, as the first footage showing so-considered exotic societies in the 1920s and 1930s was also produced to register and document their way of living (e.g., *Rituais e festas/Rituals and Feasts of Boror*, Brazil, 1916). By the 1980s and 1990s, ethnological and anthropological films focused mainly on cultural diversity and the interaction between Indigenous communities and mainstream-meshed societies.[7] Indigenous knowledge(s) were described and reported but not necessarily validated or acknowledged as complex epistemic systems, comparable to those of Western societies. Although filmmakers made a clear-cut distinction between scientific knowledge and peripheral knowledge(s), there was a consensus about the superior holistic approach that Indigenous societies had with their surrounding milieus (e.g., *Diki nima/Medicina mazateca/Mazatec Medicine*, Mexico, 1981). The onset of visual anthropology as a field prompted a reflection on the use of images as participatory instruments for the communities being depicted, instead of mere research tools.

As for fiction, from the onset of Latin American film industry, it became an appropriate arena to instill ideologies, standpoints, and ways of understanding the world. Paradigms of representation emerged responding to preconceptions, initially seeking the attention of urban audiences, mainly in the 1940s and 1950s.[8] During the next two decades, cinema ceased to be a privilege of the elites and became a form of entertainment and a platform for the dissemination of ideologies for diverse consumers. Indigenous communities became part of the audience. By the 1970s, fiction served as a medium to raise awareness among Indigenous and non-Indigenous viewers.[9] Many directors used films to remind audiences of the violence and abuse endured by native peoples, rendering cinema an important political tool (e.g., in Bolivia). This trend lasted until the 1980s when fiction became a tool to focus on individuals rather than groups. After all, democracies had been reestablished and the sense of militant need had waned. During the 1990s, narratives returned to themes revolving around ancient empires, allegorized past civilizations, and the encounter between Native Americans and Europeans. Undoubtedly, there was a link between the 500-year celebration of the "discovery" of the continent and a search for identity.

Worth emphasizing is the fact that by the beginning of the 1960s, indigeneity was already included in most formats, such as documentaries, biographies, short films, and feature films.[10] Social changes and the subsequent reestablishment of democracies influenced how Indigenous elements were depicted. Ethnical inclusion and cultural acknowledgment increased, even though oppression and abuse against disfranchised sectors of the population still took place (e.g., extractivism). Cinematic indigeneity was not any longer the exclusive domain of non-Indigenous filmmakers, but it did remain within a grid of paradigms and schemas known by audiences across Latin America. Throughout the twentieth century, cinema in the continent went through various stages led by external and internal factors, all creating a major presence of Indigenous figures and elements.[11] Indigenous cinema has consolidated its presence as a self-representational tool in the twenty-first century but remains confined to specific settings, informal networks of distribution, and a reduced number of exhibition venues.

Hegemonic channels of media production explain the relatively limited cinematic attention paid to non-Western medicinal traditions as endorsed therapeutic practices intrinsically linked to specific ecosystems and biotic factors. In Latin American cinema, historically, references to Indigenous mechanisms to restore health have been used as discursive and narrative strategies, or only briefly included. By proxy, ethnobotanical and phytopharmaceutical praxes (i.e., how the plant-related knowledge, theory, and skills are put into practice) have been majorly overlooked or framed as curiosities rather than established paradigms. Exceptions include three Mexican productions where the focus lies upon the nexus between ancestral medicine, modern times, and ecocriticism. These are the feature films *Flores en el desierto/Flowers in the Desert* (2009) and *Buenas hierbas/The Good Herbs* (2010) and the documentary film *Yacuna amor a la vida/Yacuna Love to Life* (2016). Other exceptions are not surprisingly works carried out from within Indigenous communities and inscribed in the relatively young tradition of Indigenous Cinema (e.g., *Bankilal/El hermano mayor/The Older Brother*, Mexico, 2012; *La flor que vive/*Living *Flower*, Peru, 2013; *Toyol kajal/Noosfera/Noosphere*, Mexico, 2016).

Visual culture reflects the dominancy of biomedicine and by extension the sense of clusivity (i.e., the distinction between "inclusive we" and "exclusive we") that defines how each society relates, imagines, and interacts with the notions of nature and disease. The cinematic apparatus as a materialization of technical advances and endowed with the affordances of mass communication has not been neutral in the depiction of dominant and traditional knowledge(s). As a matter of fact, at some point in history, cinema has served to frame or question with disdain the validity of ancestral therapeutic approaches.

Healer vis-à-vis Physician

From the onset of filmic representations, cinema seemed to be imbued with ideologies and stances deployed by patriarchal alignments, embodied in predominantly masculine, white characters. Variations to this convention were regarded as atypical formulations of a format conceptually monopolized and superintended by hierarchical structures. Scientific knowledge was customarily enacted by male figures who symbolically and iconically embodied the authoritativeness of science as a by-word for progress, modernity, and innovation.[12] In terms of expertise, female counterparts were more commonly intertwined with secondary roles, marginal, informal, or even scorned practices. A case in point is the figure of the respectable male doctor and parodic female Indigenous bonesetter depicted in *María Candelaria* (Mexico, 1944).

Directed by Emilio Fernández, one of the most widely screened and acclaimed films ever produced in Latin America (Grand Prix at Cannes, 1946) is a tragic love story told through the lens of disease, disavowal, and poverty.[13] At the same time, this is also a visual narrative that illustratively articulates the stereotypical ideas held about Indigenous healing methods and the ecosystems inhabited by disfranchised communities. Set in 1909, *Maria Candelaria* follows closely the romantic relationship between María (Dolores del Río) and Lorenzo Rafael (Pedro Armendáriz) and the burden of social stigma, poverty, and eventually epidemic and injustice. Their Indigenous community in the town of Xochimilco begrudgingly shuns them on the grounds that María is the daughter of a prostitute. Their position as farmers, surviving on the limited resources their small land produces, makes them vulnerable to the unscrupulous and unethical actions of Don Damian (Miguel Inclán), an influential wealthy shop owner, who is secretly and madly in love with María. Her beauty causes not only jealousy among the women of the village but also interest of an itinerant renowned painter, Pintor/Maestro (Alberto Galán), who sees María as the embodiment of an Indigenous muse.

When she falls ill from malaria, Don Damian refuses to provide the couple with any quinine that could help her fight the disease. Not seeing any other way out of this precarious situation, Lorenzo Rafael, weakened by despair, steals some of the life-saving medicine and a wedding dress, emotionally affected by María's poor health state and the impossibility of marrying her as they want to. Once Lorenzo Rafael is imprisoned, María accepts to pose for Pintor as means to retribute for the fact that he has offered to pay off the stiff amount needed to secure her lover's release from prison. Using María as a model for the facial expression and another girl as a model for the naked body parts, Pintor creates and signs his artwork, but figuratively also signs a death sentence for María. As soon as the inhabitants of Xochimilco find out about an allegedly naked image of the ostracized young girl, she is chased around and finally stoned to death. An important detail is that her last moments are not caused by malaria but by violence inflicted on her.

There are two aspects worth mentioning here. On the one hand, it is important to underline that, based on its absence from Mayan and Aztec medical books, for instance, Aztec herbals, malaria did not exist in the Americas before the arrival of Europeans.[14] In many ways, this is a reminder of the fragility of human interconnectivity on a global scale and of the undeniable shared responsibility we have toward our ecosystems at various levels. Slavery and confinement, among others, are considered as factors that facilitated the spread of the disease in the continent. There are many unanswered questions about malaria today, and even without any external interference or as by-product of European colonization, it had probably made it to the Americas anyway.[15] Yet, the path toward a future where our species is willing to face the current environmental crisis lies in recognizing that contemporary societies have already accrued enough knowledge to understand what is manageable, feasible, and preventable.

On the other hand, retrospectively, going back to *Maria Candelaria*, it is worth discussing how the eponymous character recovers from her illness (i.e., malaria) in the first place. Director Fernández presents us with a complex scenario. During the worst moments of her disease, Lorenzo Rafael fetches a *huesera*/bonesetter (Lupe del Castillo), hoping she can cure María using ancestral Indigenous medicine.[16] The bonesetter warns him that María Candelaria risks dying if she does not receive quinine. The elderly woman adds that the medicine is part of a government-implemented prophylactic and curative distribution plan—for a reason—but assures him she will come to see María nevertheless. Lorenzo Rafael ignores what audiences learn from the opening scene. The magnitude of malaria in terms of morbidity and mortality had forced mid-century Mexican authorities to deploy intensive sanitary campaigns, and quinine distribution was one attempt to eradicate the disease.[17] Hence, forcing his way into Don Damian's store is as illegal as the shop owner's attempt to prevent the young couple from receiving the medicine supplied by the state.

In the meantime, unexpectedly, a doctor (Arturo Soto Rangel) sent by Pintor has arrived. After asking some questions, the physician decides to administer María an injection once he learns that Lorenzo Rafael has given her some of the "stolen" quinine. As promised, the bonesetter arrives at the hut, carrying along all she might need to treat the patient. Indigenous healer and physician meet face to face. The conversation between them in this film from the first half of the twentieth century provides a glimpse into the set of ideas about knowledge(s) that have defined the interplay between Western and non-Western medicine for decades. Their brief interaction symbolically alludes to the embodiment of scientific knowledge and ancestral practices, the problematic technology vis-à-vis tradition dyad, biological and physiological principles in contrast with holistic treatments, and the unresolved nature-culture dilemma.

While the bonesetter warns about the danger of having a patient treated by a *matasanos* (croaker), the physician playfully asks whether a bonesetter, judging from the first part of the word (i.e., bone-), is actually an osteologist—a remark the bonesetter seems to misunderstand, except for the mocking connotation of the comment. The Indigenous healer shows signs of mistrust toward the physician and the type of modern medicine he practices. The exchange of words indicates the urban doctor is less concerned about the Indigenous practices than the bonesetter about the results of any action he could undertake to save María. They finally agree that María Candelaria will get a bone setting session with a warm ointment first and only then the treatment administered by the doctor. From a previous scene, viewers are aware that the bonesetter truly believes in the unquestionable efficacy of quinine in the treatment of malaria.[18] It becomes evident that the Indigenous healer regards her treatment as an adjunctive intervention, or as a holistic therapy she hopes will maximize the pharmacological effect of the medication.

Malaria was one of the three leading causes of death in mid-century Mexico.[19] The portrayal of the disease and its treatment, even as subplots, have left many unanswered questions, nonetheless because the film was released at a time the mosquito-borne infectious disease affected and killed thousands around the world. One might wonder about the accuracy of the time lapse between María's initial and subsequent symptoms, the mysterious content of the injection administered by the physician, and the nature of a bone massage with a warm ointment to treat a disease that develops in the liver and red blood cells. Unavoidably, the presence of the plants and the preparation of an embrocation to apply on María's body bring to mind awareness about traces of Aztec medicine. Long before Fernández's film was released, other images had served as epistemic-semiotic vehicles to communicate phytomedicinal knowledge on what to do in the case of elevation of body temperature. Figure 1.2 shows the visuality of herbs as remedies in the treatment of "excess heat" as recorded in *Libellus de Medicinalibus Indorum Herbis* (*Little Book of the Medicinal Herbs of the Indians*) (1552), also known as Badianus

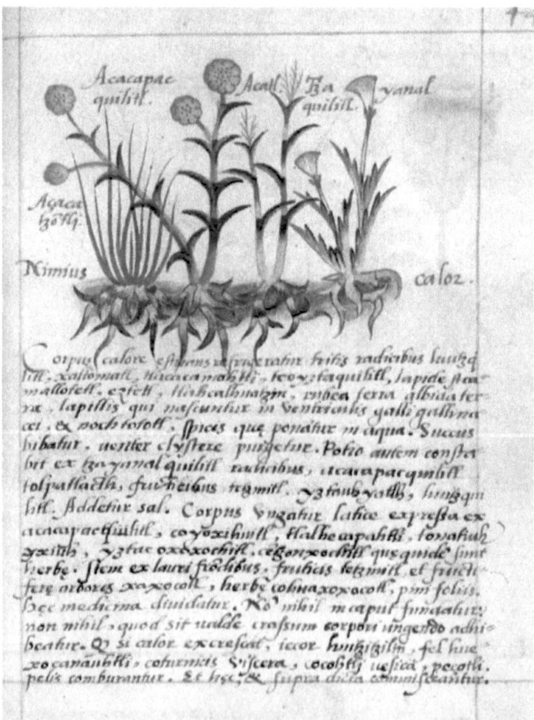

Figure 1.2 "Excessive Heat" (Folio 44r). *Source*: *Libellus de Medicinalibus Indorum Herbis* (*Little Book of the Medicinal Herbs of the Indians*)(Badianus Manuscript/Badianus Codex) (1552) by Martín de la Cruz and translated by Juan Badiano into Latin.

Manuscript by Martín de la Cruz and translated from Nahuatl into Latin by Juan Badiano.[20]

As the text reads, in the case of excess heat,

> The body is anointed with the latex squeezed from the *acapac'quuitl*, *coyo' xihuitl*, *tlahecapatli*, *tonatiuh'yxiuh*, *iztacoco-xochitl*, *centzon'oco'xochitl*, which are herbs; also using the leaves of the laurel, the bush *tetzmitl*, and the fruit trees *xa'xocotl*, the plant *cohua'xochitl*, leaves of the pine. This medicine is then divided, some poured on the head, some that is quite thick is applied as ointment on the body. (Translation by William Gates, 1939)

One can never know to which degree oral tradition and ancestral medicine inform the atmospherics in Fernández's film or inspire the filmic representation of Indigenous knowledge. It is impossible to determine if *acapac'quuitl*, *coyo' xihuitl*, *tlahecapatli*, *tonatiuh'yxiuh*, *iztacoco-xochitl*, and *centzon'oco'xochitl* are any of the plants the *huesera* intends to use to prepare the curative ointment.[21] Even if it is unintended, *María Candelaría* nevertheless draws attention to the fact that knowledge systems differ. The existence of the Badianus Codex operates as written historical evidence of Nahua medicine and which is further substantiated by the preservation of Mesoamerican therapeutic practices in present-day Central America and Mexico. In line with Mahuika's (2019) reflections, Indigenous oral tradition thrives in parallel to more hegemonic forms of knowledge transfer and production. No written sources should be needed to prove the accumulation of techniques or preservation of medicinal protocols by a community generation after generation. The fact remains that a sense of ridicule informs the portrayal of ancestral practices in Fernández's film. In regards to the Badianus Codex, Gimmel (2008) notes that the "ideal readership for the Codex did not exist at the time of its composition" and that perhaps "the ideal readers have only recently come into existence as scholars attempt to disentangle the multiple layers of meaning woven together in the Codex de la Cruz" (190). One can wonder, if, on the contrary, the ideal viewer (one who regards with disdain signs of "primitive" forms of medicine) envisioned for *María Candelaria* explains the rendering of the *huesera* and the epistemic system she represents in the film.

Biomedical perspectives are central in *María Candelaria*, aligning with a time in which Mexico is redefining itself as a modern nation willing to embrace progress through the implementation of scientifically sound policies. The figure of a derided Indigenous healer who mispronounces words in the presence of a doctor is indexical of a comparison between tradition and modernity. Fernández orchestrates a visually engaging episode that prompts viewers to question which and whose knowledge(s) should be favored when life is at stake. Xochimilco chinampas crop system, as a setting, few exchanges in Nahuatl to express agitation, and the inclusion of Mesoamerican medicinal practices are iconic reminders that Mexico's Indigenous roots are present in all aspects of daily life. Even if Fernández suggests that change involves the replacement of the old with the new, the depiction of the interaction between the community and their surroundings goes beyond an indigenist agenda. Furthermore, Fernández's popular film is also regarded as an innovative example of health communication and use of cinema as a tool to disseminate information about sanitary practices. The film subtly problematizes how hierarchies and transfers of knowledge are understood and the major implications thereof. The long history of quinine as a medicine is concomitantly a chronicle of the evolution and circulation of ethnobotanical knowledge from native communities of the Americas in the seventeenth century, imperialism and advances in chemistry in Western laboratories.[22] It is impossible to ignore that cinchona bark extracts have had pharmaceutical, political, and commercial ramifications that denote the interdependency between local knowledge(s), environment, and human health. Contextualizing the historical and scientific development of quinine as a derivative of an Andean medicinal approach is realizing that the plants brought by the bonesetter might not be so dystonic as they first appear.

María Candelaria cinematographically buttresses the realization that interconnectivity is a key factor to understand the symbiotic relation between humans and natural ecosystems. Nonetheless, because disease and cure involve biotic factors, agents, and instruments ontologically integrated into different ways according to each society's worldviews.[23] Furthermore, Fernández's acclaimed work confirms the centrality of visual culture as a repository of dominant attitudes about epistemic paradigms and the ecologies in which they are inscribed.

Diffusion, Mediation, and Acknowledgment

In August 2016, Canal TV5 Maya, the leading multilingual television channel in Guatemala, aired a special edition of *Nuestras vivencias/Our Living Experiences* on the topic of Mesoamerican medicinal practices and ancestral knowledge(s). After sharing some details about her background and expertise, the main speaker, a Kaqchikel *ajq'ij* (spiritual guide), Gloria Francisca Salazar Guaran explains how Mayan medicine has proved effective to treat life-threatening diseases, such as cancer and diabetes. Looking into the camera, she uses the opportunity to exhort viewers to trust the wisdom intergenerationally transferred, from elders and onto subsequent generations, as targeted therapies against their modern-day ailments. Answering to the questions posed by host Gabriel Armira, both in Kaqchikel and Spanish, Nana

Francisca emphasizes the importance of fusing Western and Mayan medicine to obtain the best results possible. Above all, she insists on the urgency of addressing environmental issues as means to restore health at a personal and communal level. Based on connections she makes between climate change, spiritual unrest (e.g., grudges), and pathologies of various kinds, it is easy to deduce that there is a considerable ontological divergence between the operationalization of Kaqchikel and Western therapeutical treatments.

The interview, accessible on social media platforms, can be considered as a sample of ethnographical footage and health communication, *a* type of communication, for sure. Simultaneously, it is an intimate reflection on an epistemic and epistemological system that differs from institutionalized structures that dictate how prevention, diagnosis, and treatment are to be carried out. The instrumentality and semiotic value of images not only as conveyors of information is unquestionable but also their role as sites that articulate the diversity of relations societies have with what they perceive as nature. This is particularly pertinent in the context of a short-length documentary about Nana Francisca and her role as Mayan health practitioner, released in 2020.

Directed by Guatemalan filmmakers Ana Gómez and Paola Gómez, *Rujotay k'aslemal/La vida retoñando a través de la salud/Life Sprouting through Health* delves into Nana Francisca's life and practices as an *ajq'omanela* (Mayan doctor) within a community facing major social, economic, and sanitary challenges. Set in San Antonio, Aguascalientes, the documentary, is mainly constructed in the form of a monologue and semiotically framed by visual references to objects related to the topic in question. Plants of various sizes, fire, and landscapes serve also as background for those scenes in which Nana Francisca does not interact or maneuvers the various artifacts shown in the film. Recalling passages from her own life mentioned in the abovementioned Canal TV5 interview, she explains that healers are born with the gift to cure others, progressively developed by their ability to accrue ancestral knowledge. Although anthropological sources describe *ajq'ij* as spiritual guides, Nana Francisca refers to the literal translation of the term "time counter" in order to describe her occupation and vocation. The mention of Ajaw/Ahau as the almighty creator that endows humans with their special skills shapes the tone and mode of the conversation. From a Western perspective, any allusion to supernatural forces as sources of wisdom in the context of informal educational training contradicts paradigms supported by empirical evidence, observation, and trial and error.

The materialization of Mayan cosmovision through the inclusion of statues and carved representations displayed on Nana Francisca's altar lends weight to the visual dimension of healing, as a tangible and intangible praxes. She reports using yolks and tobacco to prompt visions that allow her to make inferences about her patients' health and to interpret their symptoms. Images of lit candles, cigars, and ashes on the floor resemble the preparation of a ritual (figure 1.3) but thematically lead to Nana Francisca's remarks on the core aspect of any sickness. "The human being not only becomes physically ill, but also emotionally and energetically [ill]," she adds before proceeding to explain the connection between plants and organs, and plants and energies. A circle seems to close when the eloquent healer gives details of the connection between organs, energies, moon phases, and plant growth, suggesting liaisons and synergies not easily accommodated in Western knowledge systems.[24]

Images of what seem to be a rudimentary laboratory (according to certain benchmarks) and a rather poorly maintained greenhouse (e.g., misplaced labels) do not seem to distract the viewer from the dimension of the statements made by Nana Francisca. She shares, for instance, her dream of working closely with biomedically trained physicians, compartmentalizing the deployment of health care, on the one hand, according to spiritual and energetic paradigms (Indigenous counterpart) and, on the other, according to scientific premises (physicians). In an attempt to call for action, she reiterates the importance of raising awareness among contemporary societies about their impact on fragile ecosystems and the relation between ecological issues and human health. At this point of the documentary, any attempt to compare or relate Kaqchikel and biomedical, research-based precepts seem unproductive and futile. And yet, paradoxically, it is through an academic and science-driven consortium of researchers and doctors that Nana Francisca gained enough notoriety to draw the attention of filmmakers Ana Gómez and Paola Gómez in the first place. In fact, unbeknownst to most viewers, from a position of apparent peripherality, she is part of a group of Mayan healers who have actively been involved in synergies that seek to integrate and accommodate seemingly inconsistent

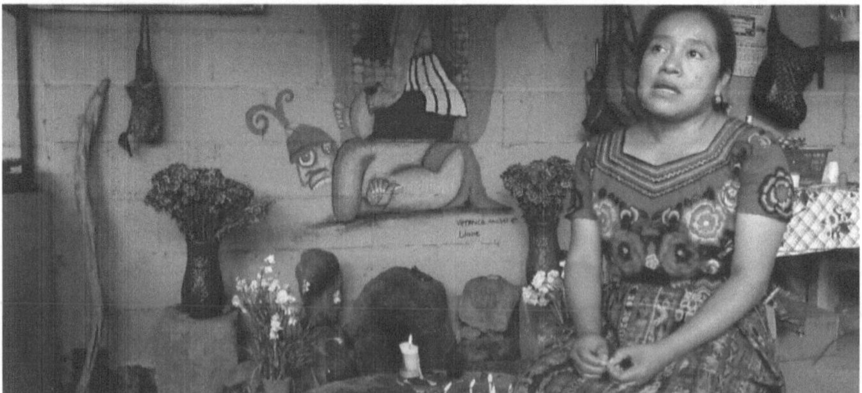

Figure 1.3 Screenshot from Documentary *Rujotay k'aslemal/La vida retoñando a través de la salud/Life Sprouting through Health* (2020).

epistemic systems. In the role of informant, Nana Francisca has indirectly collaborated and contributed to the recollection of data, eventually disseminated in ethnobotanical, phytomedicinal, and phytopharmaceutical scientific explorations. Specifically, Nana Francisca and a Council of Elders have contributed to the diffusion of Kaqchikel ethnomedicinal knowledge through their collaboration with Instituto Nacional de Cancerología / National Cancer Institute (Guatemala) and academics from the University of Valle and ETH Zurich. By proxy, she has contributed to the creation of outputs (e.g. publications) which have been mobilized across Western scientific dissemination networks.

These joint efforts have crystalized in the publication of a book on Mayan medicine (*Raxnaq'il Nuk'aslemal: Medicina Maya en Guatemala*) and recollection of data on a number of local endemic species and practices.[25] Moreover, through the lens of biomedical expertise, as it is commonly understood and disseminated in Western settings, the holistic and personalized approach of Mayan healing practices is described as an addition and a possible (potential) venue of research.[26] The overall conclusion of the body of academic literature produced as a result of this multifaceted approach to the study of ethnomedicine is that local phytomedicinal practices do have a positive impact on the patients. Although much remains to be explored, the value of documentation work lies in its possible cross-pollination among other Indigenous societies. Conclusively, the involvement of health practitioners in the family life of patients as means to guarantee general well-being is considered a practice worth replicating in similar contexts.

Notwithstanding, applying scientific rigor to the data collected through observation, analysis, and interviews, Western researchers also reach conclusions that cast doubt on certain aspects of Mayan phytomedicine. Local healers are reported to generalize at times certain conditions by labeling them as cancer, even if they are not, assigning treatments that effectively but not consistently work for inaccurately diagnosed diseases.[27] The most illuminating conclusion identified in academic papers about Mayan medicine is that its operationalization is limited, according to studies conducted so far, and that a distinction needs to be made between local and traditional Indigenous medicine.[28] One explanation for this deduction is that modern societies face a higher degree of variability/volatility of disease-causing determinants, events, and distribution compared to past sedentary and isolated communities.

Recognition of Western institutionalized scientific and scholarly knowledge production networks and agents, or lack thereof, does not mean Kaqchikel ethnomedicinal practices lose their epistemic value. The interaction of audiences with cultural externalizations mobilized through images, such as a televised interview (watched over 22,000 times) and a documentary, underlines the leverage and recognition of knowledge in all its forms. The itinerant nature of visual artifacts, embedded in spaces such as Internet repositories (e.g., YouTube), and exhibition venues, such as film festivals, secure the circulation of ideas, conceptualizations, and imaginaries at a micro- and macro-level. Mayan medicine praxis is already partly preserved in images, and it will most likely continue to be documented visually. While Cannes accelerated the distribution of *María Candelaria* (1944), in places as foreign to Mexico as Yugoslavia and former USSR, *Rujotay k'aslemal/La vida retoñando a través de la salud/Life Sprouting through Health* (2020) finds audiences, for now, in Central American screening venues (e.g., Lúdico and Icaro Film Festivals) and visual anthropology courses.

Decades apart, these two visual narratives share their involvement in documenting the diversity of perceptual relations that condition human experience biologically and topologically. A link between the specificity of knowledge and the bodies that dwell diverse geographies irrefutably prompts discussions about the rich array of meanings and interpretations of sickness, treatment, and health. Linking plants to specific organs, as Nana Francisca does, leads to considering the symbiotic significance of preserving the ecosystems where these plants actually grow. Pollution, destruction, and decimation of habitats that include organisms equated to the well-being of other organisms, from the Kaqchikel ethnomedicinal viewpoint, are utterly illogical and irresponsible. Images are not axiomatic representations of knowledge, and yet, they provide entry points into the plurality of epistemic practices observed by different cultures.

Visual externalizations replicate the multiplicity of approaches to diagnosis, treatment, and medicinal instruments. At moments of crises, they exacerbate the need to ponder about new ways of fostering, reconfiguring, or dismantling relations and dependencies. A case in point is the impact that COVID-19 has had on the communities in Aguascalientes, and specifically on the family life of Nana Francisca. A year after the onset of the pandemic, her husband Tata Paudilio Hernández, greatly affected by the infectious disease, was hospitalized, incurring medical costs the family was not able to cover. In July 2021, a fundraising raffle was organized by relatives and friends, counting on the solidarity of their local community. Images of plants were used as a centerpiece in the announcement of the charity initiative. A logical decision since the first five prizes were having access to the ethnobotany courses run by Nana Francisca, in addition to receiving medicinal products developed by her women's collective. In line with observations made by Hitziger's (2016) research team, new diseases pose a considerable challenge for those practicing traditional medicine. Visual artifacts register how societies evolve and how they cope with changes at various levels, certainly a pandemic. Cultural production has secured the mobilization of images that record the magnitude of the Coronavirus in corners of the globe overlooked by major media consortia.

As I argue in this book, each society understands the natural world differently, depending on the intimate relation communities have developed over time with their immediate surroundings at an experiential and epistemic level, without forgetting those for whom this occurs at a spiritual level. Their relation excludes those who are not conversant in the symbolic dialogue between members of a group that epistemologically agree on how to approach their habitat. Images emerge as viable tools to register this dialogue. *María Candelaria* and *Rujotay k'aslemal/La vida retoñando a través de la salud/Life Sprouting through Health* provide evidence of the sense of bioclusivity that characterizes the period of time, geographical space, and cultural realm in which they were produced. The visual healing aspect of these visual artifacts is their suitability to voice peripheral forms of knowledge and understandings about medicinal practices, forcing a recognition that there is no definite consensus on how to understand nature and the environment epistemically and ontologically. Their pictorial and semiotic presence registers collective imaginaries about health and expressions thereof through fictional and nonfictional scenarios. The human body remains central in visual culture, nonetheless because the dynamic and interplay between those on each side of the screen continuously evolve and blur, progressively expanding the repertoire of genres, cultures, and worldviews. This certainly applies to the ultimate human function that secures our survival: reproduction.

IMAGES AND ANCESTRAL SENSORIA

Births betoken the continuation of a species and this is no different for Mayan societies. A newborn is the result of months of gestation and preparation for the arrival of a human being. The process by which babies are conceived and evolve into independent organisms from their mothers is universal and relatively well understood. Yet, the conditions in which they exit the uterus vary significantly across cultures, socioeconomic contexts, and institutional settings. As historical records and cultural externalizations indicate (e.g., the DàZu sculptures or Temple of Kom Omb reliefs), midwifery is one of the oldest occupations in human history.[29] In contemporary Guatemala, *k'exel om/iyom/k'exuul/parteras/comadronas* (midwives) are as much part of the traditional medicine system as abovementioned Nana Francisca is.[30] Obstetric practices have not escaped the present-day tendency to mediatize all aspects of human life. Photojournalists, filmmakers, NGO employees stationed in the Central American nation, anthropologists working with the communities, researchers integrated into targeted projects, and other academics interested in public health are using audiovisual tools to document Mayan midwifery tradition.

The documentaries, vlogs, televised interviews, semi-staged vlogs, and filmed conversations take place in the context of a line of work poorly, if at all, recognized by Guatemalan biomedicine-trained workers and the central state. For most of the authors focusing on Mayan *parteras*, the main questions revolve around their identity, the challenges they face, and the practical and logistic dimensions of their daily activities.[31] A commonality identified in the narrations of the local midwives is how emphatical they are about their role within the communities they serve. On the one hand, they give examples of the high level of respect they enjoy among the Indigenous members living in the vicinity of their homes and which extends to the local authorities, with some reservations. On the other hand, Mayan midwives face high levels of discrimination when they attempt, for instance, to accompany patients to hospitals or be present while physicians are performing routine revisions or more complex procedures.

Perhaps due to the lack of targeted venues to disseminate videos on the topic, it is not difficult to find footage on the subject of Guatemalan midwifery on open-access platforms (e.g., YouTube). In the process, the filmed interviews serve as repositories of ancestral practices and oral tradition, otherwise not available to audiences outside the communities where the *parteras* live and work. Their comments about the mockery they experience on behalf of doctors and nurses in real life materialize also in the comments of viewers on digital platforms. Through emoticons, such as "rolling on the floor laughing emoticon", "face with tears of joy emoticon", and "grimacing face emoticon", preceded or followed by bantering and burlesque remarks, some members of the audience show signs of skepticism, perplexity, doubt, and suspicion. Some relate to the stories of the *parteras* and show tokens of support by thanking them for their commitment. It is an occupation deeply connected with the emotions of the expectant mothers, fathers, and the ones assisting them; an ancestral sensorium in the context of the heritage and epistemologies that underpin its existence. Visual culture operates as an apparatus to present the place of reproduction, pregnancy, and births within Mayan cosmovision. Through the comments left by the audiences and the high number of views—with one video surpassing over one million and a half views— it is clear that the theme intrigues and interests many spectators. A common topic mentioned by the midwives is their use of medicinal plants at all stages of their interaction with the mothers, during and after the birth has taken place. While leaves of broadleaf plantain, locally known as *llantén* (*Plantago major*), or pieces of corn silk, *xilotl/jilote* (*Stigma maydis*), can help during the recovery stages, according to the interviewed midwives, university-trained physicians tend to discredit their possible medicinal benefits.[32] One of the midwives shares with the camera an incident in which a doctor told her that, on the contrary, ethnobotanical practices increase, in fact, the mortality rates among newborns.[33] In critical scenarios, the presence of *comadronas* is specially unwanted across clinical contexts and many regret that hospital staff continuously remind them that their expertise is questionable. Through their exchanges with public health staff, *parteras* experience apprehension, disbelief, cynicism, and uneasiness about their involvement or assistance in childbearing- and parturition-related institutional contexts.[34]

Sensing a high level of dubitation and lack of trust, one *comadrona* recalls telling those present in the delivery room that her credentials lie in her position of being a *ginecóloga ancestral* (ancestral gynecologist). The interviewed *comadrona* does not provide more details about the incident. As any other spectator watching the filmed dialogue online, I cannot know the reaction of her interlocutors in that particular moment. But the fact is that maternity wards of hospitals, in most cases, observe a hierarchy structured according to qualifications in obstetrics and gynecology from accredited institutions. Only after a rigorous, highly specialized, and time-consuming training, a physician completes the requirements stipulated by health centers to engage with pregnancy, childbirth, and postpartum eventualities, at least, from a biomedical perspective.[35] From within a protocol that emphasizes on biomedicine, it is most likely that *parteras* meet apprehension and lack of collegiality. Doctors forget that "ese trabajo yo no lo inventé . . . eso viene milenarios de años [*sic*]" (I didn't make up this line of work . . . this goes back thousand of years), adds one of them. Mayan *parteras* are disappointed about the lack of recognition from health officers, nonetheless because midwives are present in many more birth than doctors in Guatemala. Some estimates indicate that between 30% and 35% of all women receive assistance of a *comadrona* during their pregnancy, parturition, or postpartum stages. Although none of the filmed midwives use the term "medicalization," they do hint at the fact that, for most part of human history, mothers have not given birth in hospital settings. In a peeved tone of voice, a Mayan *comadrona* asks: "¿Quién atendió al doctor? . . . Una comadrona" (Who delivered the doctor? . . .A midwife). For the sake of the expectant women, it saddens them not to be able to collaborate with physicians in order to achieve the best possible results for mothers and newborns.

Data gathered from diverse sources and for different purposes confirm the important part of ancestral midwives in assisting pregnant women, both in urban and rural contexts.[36] Their visual presence in videos posted on social media platforms and subsequent responses only reflect a fraction of their actual presence in the healthscapes of Guatemalan child-bearing women. At a social level, *comadronas* also fulfill positions not necessarily filled by other health professionals or state-run institutions. In the films, mothers (or patients, depending on the definition of pregnancy being used) share their first-hand experience giving birth to children under the supervision of local *parteras*. Intimacy, involvement, attachment, concern, and personal care are the terms used by the interviewed women and men. Some explain that while hospital staff cannot cope with full delivery rooms where each woman is merely a number, midwives become part of the family throughout the gestation process. A relationship as, one of the fathers explains, that remains long after the baby is born and to the extent that children call the midwife that delivers them "abuela" (grandmother) when they meet them in the street. The midwives sharing their stories attribute this attachment to their engagement in creating "un parto humanizado" (a humanized birth) and evidence that they do not go to school to *learn* how to deliver babies, they are born to be *parteras.* In this regard, some share the difficulties they face doing a line of work that sometimes disrupt their private lives, to the degree, that it has affected negatively their own marriages.

As explained by the interviewed midwives, Mayan *parteras* receive their gift to help others to give birth from Ajaw/Ahau (creator). Although some are grateful for the recent attempts on behalf of local and central governments to offer them training opportunities and more acknowledgment for their role within the informal health system of the country, *comadronas* explain this is their *samaj* (pre-assigned labor).[37] Connections between the *nawal* (spirit/energy) of each one of them, along with their *q'ij* (birthday), in their words, is enough accreditation for them to gain recognition about their vocation from their community. While the cameras register the facilities where so many women have come for assistance during their pregnancy, one *k'exelom* comments on the paradoxical aspects of being put in this world to deliver babies. "Es un don y una maldición" (it is a gift and a curse), she utters. The lack of recognition from formal institutions weighs heavy, but none of the interviewed midwives seems reluctant or hesitant to continue serving the community. After four decades, one *partera* notes, things are changing and becoming more difficult. Changes in lifestyles result in more complex births. The Coronavirus pandemic has also had a toll on their daily interaction with the pregnant women living in isolated parts of the country. Even if the midwives' labor might meet incredulity and hesitancy among spectators, particularly from a scientific perspective, the images show the actual circumstances in which some of the births take place. "Tengo mi linterna" (I have a flashlight), explains an *iyom*, aware that this can be a vital tool in case she faces the challenge of delivering a newborn during the evening in a home deprived of electricity. The visual sensorium of the footage used for the interviews rests in its capacity to draw attention to women and men working for the sake of securing the health and life of two individuals (mother and child), jeopardizing at times their own.

One strand that unites *María Candelaria, Raxnaq'il Nuk'aslemal: Medicina Maya en Guatemala*, and the series of filmed interviews with Mayan midwives reviewed in this chapter is the use of visual productions to mediate messages about the care and cure of the body. Assisted by cameras and those maneuvering them, these medicine women participate in promoting therapeutical and healing practices coherent with their own sense of bioclusivity. While in fiction (*María Candelaria*), the traditional healer advises about the use of quinine (state-of-the-art knowledge at the time), in real-life scenarios, Nana Francisca and a cohort of *parteras* share with viewers what they believe contributes to lead disease-free lives or to start one in the best way possible. Images frame, register, archive, and broadcast the understanding of those being filmed, either scripted or unscripted. Through optical and editorial processes, ideas about the role of nature in the pursuit of health materialize in audiovisual artifacts. They remain evidence of the various ways in which societies at large and individuals regard the *natura-Homo sapiens* dynamic in the context of health. At the same time, these epistemic-semiotic artifacts inscribe themselves in the history of Mesoamerican medicine, confirming that knowledge systems materialize through various media and formats. A sixteenth-century manuscript and YouTube homemade interview can both disseminate knowledge.

NOTES

1. Ezra (2006).
2. Gonzalez Rodriguez (2022).
3. The establishment of *Pueblos de Indios* remains an exception to colonial endeavors to disintegrate the social tissue of established communities in order to weaken their political status (Ouweneel, 2018).
4. On the bloodletting tradition described by Wafer in what is today Panama, Ortiz de Montellano (1990) has observed that it was possibly part of cause-effect healing practice. The cause, blood built up in the brain that led to headaches, the effect, needed to be treated, according to this local etiological approach, by releasing blood. Bloodletting has been identified as a curative method in many parts of the world (e.g., ancient Egypt and Greece) and in pre-Columbian America, Seggiaro (1969) asserts almost all native nations practiced it in one way or another. The full passage from Lionel Wafer's book *The New Voyage and Description of the Isthmus of America* (1699): "On this Hill live Fifty Principal Men of the Country, all under Lacentas Command, who is as a Prince over all the South part of the Isthmus of Darien; the Indians both there and on the North side also, paying him great respect. But the South side is his Country, and this Hill his Seat or Palace. There is only one Canoa belonging to it, which serves to ferry over Lacenta and the rest of them. When we were arrived at this Place, Lacenta discharged our Guides, and sent them back again, telling us. That 'twas not possible for us to Travel to the North side at this Season; for the Rainy Season was now in its height, and Travelling very bad; but told us we should stay with him, and he would take care of us. And we were forc'd to comply with him. We had not been long here before an Occurrence happen'd,

which tended much to the increasing the good Opinion Lacenta and his People had conceiv'd of us, and brought me into particular Esteem with them. It so happen'd, that one of Lacenta's Wives being indisposed, was to be let Blood; which the Indians perform in this manner. The Patient is seated on a Stone in the River, and one with a Bow shoots htde Arrows into the naked Body of the Patient, up and down; shooting them as fast as he can, and not mi';';irio; any part. But the Arrows are gaged, so that they penetrate no farther than we generally thrust our Lancets. And if by chance they hit a Vein which is full of Wind, and the Blood spurts out a htde, they wiU leap and skip about, shewing many Antick Gestures, by way of rejoycing and triumph. I was by while this was performing on Lacenta' s Lady, and, perceiving their Ignorance, told Lacenta, That if he pleased, I and that man that is out of favor had as good be out of his wife Lacenta seems to have been a Chief Paramount over smaller chieftains or heads of clans; the same custom prevails among the Cuna of the San Bias territory to-day, the Nele of Aligandi, for example, receiving respect from the ad- jacent tribes, each with its family chief or sagila, would shew him a better way, without putting the Patient to so much Torment. Let me see, says he; and at his Command, I bound up her Arm with a piece of Bark, and with my Lancet breached a Vein. But this rash attempt had like to have cost me my Life. For Lacenta seeing the Blood issue out in a Stream, which us'd to come only drop by drop, got hold of his Lance, and swore by his Tooth, that if she did otherwise than well, he would have my Heart's Blood. I was not moved, but desired him to be patient, and I drew off about 12 Ounces, and bound up her Arm, and desired she might rest till the next Day, by which means the Fever abated, and she had not another Fit" (Wafer, 1699) (This book is in the public domain).

5. Van Groesen (2012).

6. Gonzalez Rodriguez (2022).

7. Ginsburg (2011).

8. Gonzalez Rodriguez (2022).

9. Jorge Sanjinés, for instance, develops a special vocabulary that challenges established political hierarchies, even if his productions include exoticist elements (Wood, 2006).

10. Mateus Mora (2012).

11. D'Argenio (2022).

12. Several studies have been conducted on the figure of the male doctor in mediatic representations, see, for instance, Carson and Llewellyn-Jones (2000), Harper and Moor (2005), and Gustafsson (2014).

13. Grand Prix was the name of the highest prize awarded in Cannes from 1939 to 1954 and from 1964 to 1974, intermittently and eventually replaced by Palme D'Or.

14. See Emmart (1935), Ortiz de Montellano (1975), Tucker and Janick Flora (2019), Reyes-Chilpa et al. (2021), and Schendel (2021).

15. Hall and Tamïr (2022).

16. On the concept of *hueseros* and their role within Mexican health landscape, see Navaroo Campos, Peña Sánchez, and Maya (2017); Campo (2018).

17. Gómez-Dantés and Birn (2000).

18. A scenario that would align with the outreach of intensive malaria-related educational campaigns to eradicate malaria (Cueto, 2007).

19. Gómez-Dantés and Birn (2000).

20. The full translation of Folio 44r by Gates (1939): "Excessive heat The body when overheated is relieved by the ground roots of the huitzquilitl, xahtomatl, tlaca'camotli, teoHztaquilitl, the stone a'camollotetl, the eztetl, tlacal'huatzin, red earth, white earth, and the stones found in the stomachs of a cock and the noch'totl, with sharp stones, all then put in water. This is drunk and the abdomen purged with a clyster. A potion is also prepared from tzayanal'quilitl roots, the acacapac'quilitl, tol'patl' ctli, the bushes tetzmitl, iztauhyauh, huitz'quilitl, with added salt. The body is anointed with the latex squeezed from the acapac'quuitl, coyo' xihuitl, tlahecapatli, tonatiuh'yxiuh, iztacoco-xochitl, centzon'oco'xochitl, which are herbs; also using the leaves of the laurel, the bush tetzmitl, and the fruit trees xa'xocotl, the plant cohua'xochitl, leaves of the pine. This medicine is then divided, some poured on the head, some that is quite thick is applied as ointment on the body. If the heat rises, take the blood of the huitzitzilin, the gall of the huexo'canauhtli, the viscera of a quail, bladder of the cocotli, skin of the pezotli, burned together. These and the above are to be mixed together." Since there are some difference, I am including Emmart's (1940) translation: "Excessive heat. A body sweltering with heat is cooled with the ground roots of huitzquiltl, xaltomatl, tlacacamohtli, and teoyztaquilitl; the stone of acamal-lotetl, eztetl, and tlahcalhuatzin; red earth; white earth; the stones which grow in the stomach of the rooster and nochtototl; and grain which are to be put into water. The juice is to be drunk, and the abdomen purged with a clyster. A potion, moreover, will consist of tzayanalquilitl roots, acacapacquilitl, tolpatlactli, and the shrubs etzmitl, yztauhyatlh, and huitzquilitl. Salt is to be added. The body is to be anointed with the sap expressed from acacapacquilitl, coyoxihuitl, tlalhecapahtli, tonatiuhyxiuh, yzta-coxoxochitl, and centzonxochitl, all of which are plants. Likewise from the fronds of laurel, of the shrub tetzmitlo, and of the fruit tree xaxocotl, from the herb cohuaxoxo-cotl, and from pine needles. This medicine is to be divided: some is to be poured on the head; some, which is very thick, is to be used for anointing the body. But if the heat rises, the liver of huitzitzilin, the gall bladder of huexocnauhtli, the viscera of quail, the bladder of cocohtli, and the skin of peçotli are to be burned. And these and the things mentioned above are to be mixed."

21. In their systematic study, Tucker and Janick (2020) enlist the various processes of previous and present identification, geographical distribution and uses of these plants in modern-day contexts.

22. Crawford (2016), Heaton (2018), and Christensen (2021) explore various aspects of the use of cinchona in colonial settings.

23. In line with findings from qualitative interviews discussed in chapters 3 and 5, cultural outputs are assessed based on their capacity to echo the epistemologies and lived experiences of the viewers/audiences.

24. A close example found in the history of medicine includes the doctrine of signatures that suggests that morphological characteristics of plants are indexical of their therapeutic properties and value, or anthropomorphized in the pursuit of patterns that explain the natural world (Buchanan, 1938; Torshin, 2007; Wen, 2022).

25. Although, in the context of Hayden's (2005) discussion of the representational dilemma of "traditional knowledge," it is difficult to assess what a publication like this actually tells us about North-South collaborations. Even if Hayden focuses in her discussion mainly on medicinal plants, she insightfully invites us to think "how are notions of comparative efficacy being re-calibrated with the promise of benefit-sharing (and its ever-present twin, the accusation of biopiracy) on the horizon?" (197).

26. Hitziger (2016).

27. Barrios (2017).

28. Hitziger (2016).

29. Graham (1951).

30. The occupation midwife has different translations according to the language spoken in each linguistic community. The Spanish words *comadrona* (or less used partera) are encompassing terms, used widely in the country, but mainly linked to the mestizo populations. Other terms are *iloneel tuuj* (Achi), *sik`om unin* (Akateko), *xu`yum / xi`iyum* (Awakateko), *xi`iyom* (Chalchiteko), *ajk`ojb`/ ajk'ot na'k / irna`k* (Cho`orti`), *ik`um el unin* (Chuj), *agüdahatu* (Garifuna), *ixnana'chich* (Itza), *k`uyintxa`* (Ixil), ilom (Jakalteko/Popti'), *iyom* (K`iche`), *yoq`il / b`etx`lon* (Mam), *ix paatz'*(Mopan), *ahk`ulul Xilu`* (Poqomam), *ajilool / ajloq`ool /* ilool/ loq`ol *ha`lak`un / k'ulul ha'lak'un / molol ha'lak'un* (Poqomchi`), *sik'om unin* (Q`anjob`al), *aj xokol k`uula`al* (Q`eqchi`), *ajtuuj* (Sakapulteko), *akjkuun* (Sipakapense), *yoq'ol* (Tektiteko), *iiyoom* (Tz`utujil and Uspanteko), *müyalhatahana* (Xinka) (Ministerio de Salud Pública y Asistencia Social, 2015 / ALMG, 2015).

31. Since it is impossible to protect the identity of the interviewed mothers shown in the films, I have decided to restrain from providing the specific names of the corpus of videos reviewed in this chapter of the book.

32. There seems to be scientific evidence that *Plantago major* has medicinal properties, in particular in terms of anti-inflammatory properties, as mentioned by the interviewed midwives (Núñez et al., 1997; Gomez-Flores, 2000; Türel et al. 2009; Nazarizadeh et al., 2013; Reina, 2013; Hussan, 2015; Adom, 2017). In vitro and in vivo (e.g., on rodents) pharmacological studies and experiments indicate *Stigma maydis* shows sign of bioactive properties that include effective diuretic agents, substantiating the practices observed by one of the interviewed *iyoms*. Antibacterial effects are nevertheless effective to certain types of small single-celled organisms (Alam, 2011). Furthermore, scientific publications shed light on the vast geographical distribution of the practice of using *Stigma maydis* for urinary tract conditions (e.g., in China) (Hasanudin, 2012; Saheed at al., 2015; Zhang et al., 2015; Jeong et al., 2017; Birla and Dwivedi, 2020).

33. For more on the medicinal plants used by midwives, see Cominsky (Appendix I, 2021).

34. There are certainly risks involved in not having access to obstetricians and gynecologists in cases of emergency. Berry (2006) observes that there are issues with a not so successful referral-based system, mainly because of the *iyoma*'s (*iyoma* is the plural form of *iyom*) and pregnant women's understanding of their births. In general, "Most women would rather wait until a problem manifests to be referred to the hospital than to needlessly sacrifice the quality of their birth experience" (1969).

35. As stipulated by Edict 90-97 (Decreto Número 90-97, Código de Salud – CICAD) in Guatemalan Health Code (Congreso de Guatemala,1997).

36. As Hinojosa (2004), Schooley et al. (2009), Chary et al. (2013), Cosminsky (2021) conclude. This does not seem to be the case only in Guatemala. An extensive body of scholarly knowledge has explored the versatile role of midwives within the communities where they operate and its extend beyond obstetric assistance or gestation-related issues. Overviews of the cases of Brazil (Gualda et al., 2012), Costa Rica (Jenkins, 2001), Iran (Bahadoran et al., 2009), Kenya (Dawson et al., 2015), Papua New Guinea (Sadiv and Allan, 2018), Thailand (Liblub et at., 2020), and The Netherlands (Benoit et al., 2005) provide insights about the heterogeneousness of midwifery at the nexus between health, gender identity, and individualized care.

37. Through a legislation passed in 2015, the Guatemalan state has included midwifery as a line of work recognized, supervised, and supported according to four stipulations: "Government Agreement (Number 102-2015). Guatemala, March 16, 2015. Article 1. Approval: The National Policy for Midwives of the Four Peoples of Guatemala is approved: Maya, Garifuna, Xinca and Mestizo, formulated by the Ministry of Public Health and Social Assistance in coordination with the organizations of midwives, and will be applicable throughout the national territory. Article 2. Coordination: The Healthcare Unit for Indigenous Peoples and Interculturality of the Ministry of Public Health and Social Assistance will be the entity responsible for preparing the action plan and coordinating the implementation of the National Policy for the National Policy of Midwives of the Four Peoples of Guatemala: Maya, Garifuna, Xinca and Mestizo, coordinating and facilitating actions between the different public and private institutions that correspond to guarantee compliance with the same. Article 3. Financing: The Ministry of Public Health and Social Assistance will allocate the respective budget for the financing of the related national policy, who may sign cooperation agreements with national and international cooperation organizations that ensure compliance with the human rights of women and maternal neonatal health. Article 4. Interinstitutional Relations: The public institutions that have attributions and functions related to the issue must effectively comply with the National Policy of Midwives of the Four Peoples of Guatemala: Maya, Garifuna, Xinca and Mestizo. For this purpose, the aforementioned institutions must coordinate their actions with the Healthcare Unit for Indigenous Peoples and Interculturality of the Ministry of Public Health and Social Assistance." Original text in Spanish: "Acuerdo Gubernativo. Número 102-2015. Guatemala, 16 de marzo de 201. Artículo 1. Aprobación: Se aprueba la Política Nacional de Comadronas de los Cuatro Pueblos de Guatemala: Maya, Garifuna, Xinca y Mestizo, formulada por el Ministerio de Salud Pública y Asistencia Social en coordinación con las organizaciones de comadronas, la cual será de aplicación en todo el territorio nacional. Artículo 2. Coordinación: La Unidad de Atención de la Salud de los Pueblos Indígenas e Interculturalidad del Ministerio de Salud Pública y Asistencia Social, será la ente responsable de elaborar el plan de acción y coordinar la implementación de la Política Nacional de Política Nacional de Comadronas de los Cuatro Pueblos de Guatemala: Maya, Garifuna, Xinca y Mestizo, coordinando y facilitando las acciones entre las diferentes instituciones públicas y privadas que corresponda para garantizar el cumplimiento de la misma. Artículo

3. Financiamiento: El Ministerio de Salud Pública y Asistencia Social, asignará el presupuesto respetivo para el financiamiento de la política nacional relacionada , quién podrá suscribir convenios de cooperación con organizaciones nacionales y de cooperación internacional que velen por el cumplimiento de los derechos humanos de las mujeres y la salud materno neonatal. Artículo 4: Relaciones Interinstitucionales. Las instituciones públicas que tengan atribuciones y funciones relacionadas con el tema deberán dar efectivo cumplimiento a la Política Nacional de Comadronas de los Cuatro Pueblos de Guatemala: Maya, Garifuna, Xinca y Mestizo. Para el efecto, las referidas instituciones deberán coordinar sus acciones con la Unidad de Atención de la Salud de los Pueblos Indígenas e Interculturalidad del Ministerio de Salud Pública y Asistencia Social" (Public announcement printed in national newspapers, Ministerio de Salud Pública y Asistencia Social, 2015).

Chapter 2

Animated Epistemologies

Beliefs, attitudes, and worldviews are expressed through the representation and materiality of imaginaries that mirror cultural stances, circumstantially educational and ludic, and yet, often equally political and commercial. If knowledge is an assemblage of conceptualizations, cognitive processes, awareness, familiarity, assumed facts, and understandings, the corpus of study of this chapter—toys, children's books, animated media content, and medical philately—can be considered to be epistemological receptacles and, in light of their pedagogic potentiality, epistemological amplifiers. In societies where access to technology and mass-produced artifacts is common, illustrations operate as vehicles to communicate knowledge, used in private and public settings as part of the larger enterprise of educating and communicating. As this chapter shows, the natural world and its medicinal properties can be detected in the visual composition of, for instance, a televised animated series and a postage stamp. These too are hosts of cultural tropes intentionally wrapped in chromatically appealing formats. As trivial and small as a toy can be, for instance, it still reflects the networks of design, production, marketing, and circulation behind its existence, and more importantly, even if minimally, it encapsulates notions about its own place within the system of knowledge of its creators.

TOYING WITH HEALTH AND NATURE

Children are not immune to the circulation of visual representations that convey ideas about the interplay between nature, health, and culture. Illustrative representations and playful objects operate as didactic tools or at least as repositories of ideas that societies pass on to the next generation. Being conversant in the language of images is an unavoidable part of a process of enculturation, nonetheless in the pictorially invasive twenty-first century. From an early age, exposure to visual and ludic artifacts occurs in one way or another. Toys are examples of cultural artifacts that seductively materialize a reflection of their producing societies. They offer children, and adults as well, the possibility of learning about their surroundings, imagining one that does not exist, and experiencing the co-creation of a parallel reality. Engaging with a miniature version of objects designed by grownups is nevertheless interacting with the set of values that inform their conceptualization, for instance, about nature and the care and cure of the body. Archeological findings indicate toys have accompanied children since time immemorial, and in one format or another, they appear to be universal. Archeological work done in all corners of the globe points out the universality of toys. While Park (1998) explores, for instance, children's playful artifacts in Inuit societies, de Maret (2016) shows the interplay between the information provided by the tenth-century Kisalian graves and contemporary practices of informants in the present-day Democratic Republic of Congo. Toys are central to a survey about ludic material culture in Late Antiquity and Byzantium.[1] Moreover, a study about figurines—some depicting clothes still worn today by children and women in extreme North Siberia (e.g., fur coveralls/*kerkery*)—provides insights into the life of children in an Ice Age context.[2]

Acknowledgment of childhood as a stage in the human development with specific needs and practices, prompted by changes in attitudes and economic progress, has furthermore facilitated the commercialization of toys as an industry.[3] Expansion and diversification of products targeted at children are linked to economic interests as much as they are to cultural repertoires, popular culture, trends, stereotypes, and gender-oriented assumptions. Action figures, formerly known as boy dolls, are an example of a toy that emerged as an attempt to increase profits while adhering to culture-conditioned understandings of masculinity and femininity.[4] Launching a product that would attract the interest of young boys involved rebaptizing and reconceiving the concept of dolls, and today action figures are some of the most popular toys among children.[5] A tradition initiated by the appearance of an army figurine in 1964 has evolved through the decades, reflecting shifting ideological attitudes, historic events, and understandings of daily practices, occupations, knowledge systems, and beliefs.

The stark contrast between, for example, assumptions about Western and non-Western medicine transcends into the world of the Lego minifigures, which it is worth mentioning, have been iconic action figures since their first debut in 1975.[6] Released at different times, slightly adapted in the context of various themes, and paying attention to important changes, such as gender emancipation, there are many versions of minifigures that represent occupations carried out by health professionals. All along, the symbolic value of white and blue robes, similar to those that distinguish the scientists figurines, is indexical of the connection between health-oriented professions and the domains of science. Besides the expected uniforms worn by doctors, surgeons, nurses, paramedics, and equipment operators that make them recognizable, minifigure fans have at their disposition complementary accessories, such as miniature syringes and scissors. Figurines that represent biomedicine-related occupations are available only in thematic settings that are imagined to take place in the present and, in geographical venues, best identified as parts of the Western world.

For other dimensions or times, medicine is either not relevant or perhaps carried out by a character that personifies the acquisition of knowledge at the time. For instance, while a castle cannot dispense with a jester, it is the figure of the wizard, available in good and evil versions, who could at best epitomize the existence of a body of knowledge about health and disease in premodern times. Far away from medieval Europe, or in the modern settings, what could be contemporary Denmark—Lego is based in Billund, after all—the Wild West looks quite different, according to the Western thematic lines released in 1997 and 2002. Health concerns of the *Indians*, as the encompassing thematic sub-name reads, are in the hands of the Indian Medicine Man. A figurine that only comes in a male version and does not seem to need a specific set of tools. There are nevertheless some accessories at his disposal, which include black spiders, neon-colored flames, and irregularly shaped cacti.

Indian Medicine Man wears a buffalo horn headdress, painted beadwork, and traditional regalia, which emphatically differs from the printed stethoscope, thermometer, and pencil that complement the attire of the physician figurine. Compared to the other Native American statuettes of the same thematic line, his attire is rather austere. Medicine Man wears a coat ornamented with two round-shaped emblems and a fringed breechclout decorated with a belt. The complexity of the painting on his face adds a sense of status and mysticism. While the minifigures of the City Hospital thematic line display Stars of Life accentuated by the Rod of Asclepius, the Medicine Man features two feathers and a laced coat. The lack of instruments of any kind for someone whose occupation is to heal the community intuitively suggests that his methods and approaches differ from those deployed by the physicians working in hospitals and in urban areas.[7]

His community is much smaller and consists only of an Indian chief, an Indian female, and other figures collectively known as Indians, but distinguishable by the color of their shirts or whether they carry a quiver. The prototypical Western setting is further inhabited by a cohort known as cowboys and which includes figurines of a banker, gold prospectors, bandits, cavalry colonels, cavalry lieutenants, and cavalry soldiers. Stereotypes lie at the core of the representation of the members of each community, their roles, and the possible combinations of scenarios and situations that could emerge from their interaction, based on who they epitomize, and the characteristics each one of them embodies.[8] The visuality of ethnicity intermingles with the pictoriality of cultural traits and externalizations in its various forms.[9]

The power of dissemination of ideas through toys is easily overlooked, but it is not child's play, at least not entirely. Despite their size, two 4.28 gram action figures, such as the Surgeon and Medicine Man statuettes, have nevertheless the capacity to illustrate and elucidate some of the tensions between dominant approaches to science, epistemic regimes, and imaginaries about which knowledge(s) are to be recognized as valid and which not. Drawing a parallel between the figurines that depict Western and non-Western medicine—even if they are supposedly situated in a Wild *West* setting—indicates that healing and health are portrayed to be morphologically and semiotically entwined with the geographies and the peoples who inhabit those spaces. The presence of a surgeon, doctor, nurse, and paramedic evocatively conveys the notion that biomedicine is characterized by a stablished hierarchy, degrees of specialization, and a connection with other epistemic practices. The emblematic lab coats visually bridge biomedicine and science. The Lego figurines become objects that educate about the operationalization of modern-day health systems and, for many, even objects of self-identification, for instance, for children of health professionals. As engaging and inspiring as they can be, the minifigures however do suggest Indigenous medicine is practiced empty-handed with a kind of knowledge only suitable for men, and which is nevertheless necessary, nonetheless because of the presence of armed bandits and a potential conflict between Native Americans and non-Indigenous communities.[10] Indian Medicine Man is not only the toy version of an archetype but also the solidification of an assumption about the epistemic systems of an Indigenous Other, enchanting and interesting, but different and foreign.

Toys are as material as they are visual and, hence, have a significance in terms of views and circulation of stereotypes and abstractions about science, technology, and the natural world. Due to the stage in life in which these objects play a special role in the cognitive development and learning strategies of their users, they retain a sense of referentiality.[11] In the case of the Lego action figures, the creation of each character is dictated by the inclusion of elements that can tap into children's play repertoires. Each figurine seeks to reflect the essence of whatever ritual, activity, or purpose for which it stands. As much as Lego minifigures encourage the imagination of younger generations, in the process, they nevertheless perpetuate fixed preconceptions about, among others, ethnicity, gender roles, occupations, and habits.[12] While in the imagined Middle Ages, for instance, the use of swords congruently aligns with the use of horses, in the City thematic line, syringes coherently match with the deployment of paramedic helicopters. It is not clear to which extent children wonder about the mutability of the human body and needs throughout the ages, although they probably do. Be that as it may, except for the wizard figurine, the absence of any form of physician in medieval times might coincide with narratives about magical potions, spells, and witchcraft. Alternatively, in modern-day thematic settings, the presence of medical staff with instruments visually constructed to imply advances in technology and complex equipment denotes that their clinical practices are not based on spiritual, otherworldly, or theurgic curative techniques. The diversity of archetypes through figurines is complemented with a variety of environments in which the stories allegedly unfold.

By producing portrayals of *distant* geographies and their peoples through the materiality of statuettes, Lego unavoidably offers an interpretation of the interaction other societies have with their surroundings. Snake Charmer minifigure is an example thereof. It is a piece carefully ornamented with a bead necklace, a gold pendant, a white turban, and a curly moustache as black as the noticeably bushy eyebrows that give him an expression of astonishment. As with other action figures, the vividness of colors is strategic. Snake Charmer wears a lime green shirt that highlights his intensely white pants.[13] Optional and quite logical accessories include a cobra flute and an elapid snake in an upward position, displaying a hood formed by its flaps. In common with Indian Medicine Man, the Snake Charmer does not exist in a feminine version, which probably implies these are not occupations imagined to be carried out by women, or that these are métiers that require a specific talent, or a gift, assumed to be most likely possessed by men.[14] Another reading is that these appointments are related to a special status in the parts of the world where they are carried out and to how women are perceived *there*.

A narrative of otherness informs the inclusion of references to nature in the world of the Lego minifigures, at least, from a geographical and cultural perspective. The spatiality of tropicalism in the universe of these Danish action figures is built on blocks that can be arranged figuratively and literally to reanimate scenarios endowed with colonialist and imperialist undertones while retaining a sense of playfulness and entertainment. Although the attire of the Jungle Explorer and Wildlife Photographer figurines suggests special equipment is needed to encounter other types of topologies, the thematic line Jungle Exploration Site is actually the materialization of an undisclosed tropic corner of the planet, according to long-standing European precepts. Probably inspired by the Age of Exploration, as the promotional video suggests, the main goal is to extract a treasure hidden inside a dilapidated stone temple, register new discoveries, and survive the challenges of the tropics.

Wilderness does present a problem to the urban team of experts in charge of the dangerous mission even if leopards, snakes, crocodiles, and giant spiders enhance the inhospitable character of this tropical location. The dichotomy between tradition and modernity is epitomized by the suggested sketch of the temple children are encouraged to build and that has served as a vault for a particular type of golden frog statue. The structure of the ruins and the sculpturing tradition indicate this was (or is) the home of a local civilization, also undisclosed. Despite the risks it involves, jewels of various colors and shapes make an expedition to this part of the globe even more profitable, significantly mitigated by the level of expertise of the explorers and their special equipment.

City Jungle Helicopter Pilots, City Jungle Explorers, and City Jungle Engineer of both genders are geared up with everything they might need to succeed. The tools and gadgets drawn on their torso, or sets of accessories attachable to their C-shaped empty hands, enhance the body of knowledge, set of skills, training, and experience their occupation names imply. City Jungle Scientist female and male statuettes furthermore confirm the role and importance of science in a mission that demands mastery and dexterity in order to make sense of an unknown territory. Identifiable by their white lab coats, colored glasses, test tubes, and measurement equipment, the scientist minifigures reinforce the idea that each society has its own epistemic practices. Along with the engineers, these figures emblematically tap into concepts, such as scientific method, technology, and discoveries; even if science is probably a completely unknown practice to the young Lego fans.

An old hardly legible wrinkled map confirms this is not the city where the team normally lives, quite the opposite, a location that needs to be conceptualized, understood, and charted if the explorers dare to do so. As the promotional video implies, players are encouraged to use some of the pieces and building blocks to recreate the scene of a crashed plane and place it on top of the temple, adding an element of suspense and adventure to the Jungle Exploration site. The smashed unmanned aircraft enhances the sense that others have attempted to explore this area before, without success. A box containing gems, expected to be staged by players as if it emerged from the abandoned fuselage, is meant to provide cues about the previous explorers. A photograph camera, measurement equipment, and test tubes containing a blue and a green substance indicate the mission has a scholar scope.

Nature is presented as a phenomenon worth understanding, observing, and documenting, as much as respecting in terms of dangers and life-threatening situations. Wild animals present challenges the explorers are expected to address with care. As an extension in subsequent editions of the jungle thematic setting, Lego has added new pieces that furthermore strengthen the notion that this tropical paradise can also be unwelcoming and harsh, such as a machete and caricaturized oversized Venus flytrap (*Dionaea muscipula*). All evidence suggests this is an uninhabited forgotten location. Remains of a presumably ancient culture, in the form of valuable golden statues and precious stones, are an unclaimed treasure probably because they do not belong to anyone. Any finding or discovery for scientific purposes is hence part of a collection of data that could be imagined to enrich knowledge in fields such as archeology, biology, history, and zoology. Artifacts extracted from the ruins, one could assume, are destined to appear in museums and national galleries, after being studied and investigated for the advancement of humanity.

Human history, even if children playing with Lego action figures are unaware of this fact, has taught us that there are other possible scenarios or outcomes related to this type of exploration. The temple and what is to be found inside might actually be located in a territory inhabited by a community uninterested in extracting objects from it or perhaps in keeping them inside as they might have a symbolic value that escapes or is not relevant to the Jungle City explorers. The abandoned ruin could as well be a tomb, meant to not be entered, and which might explain the trap mechanism devised in one of the watchtowers, showing Lego designers acknowledge exploration can at times also mean trespassing. Fantasizing with the idea of exploring no man's land sounds, in many ways, as a quite adventurous endeavor, except if one remembers, again, what human history can teach us about journeys into unknown territories for the sake of economic, political, and scientific projects. No jungle or corner of the globe is really entirely empty or has no community who claims its ownership. Cultural representations that advance the idea of a place where local populations can imaginatively be erased from their own lands for the sake of an entertaining narrative, even from the harmless situatedness of a child's toy uncomfortably resonate with a necropolitical rhetoric.[15] Lego thematic lines are destined for children and, yet, seen through the lens of historic awareness, an exploration into the jungle with boxes to be filled with gems does lead to some unsavory connections and references. The practice of venturing into far-flung corners of the globe and extracting artifacts somehow overlaps with the paternalistic and imperialist tradition of ransacking, plundering, and commercializing items that, decontextualized from their sites of production, become commodities. By the same token, the test tubes held by the scientist figurines, even if they are colorful and ornamental, slightly alert about the risks of bioprospecting programs.[16] Projects engrained in the articulation of systems tightly defined, today as in the eighteenth-century New World-Old World context, by factors that push scientific endeavors toward and away from "certain parts of nature" and identified by Schiebinger (2004) as "funding priorities, global strategies, national policies, the structures of scientific institutions, trade patterns, and gender politics" (226).

The idea of a jungle as a source of raw materials for pharmaceuticals remains unchanged and is paradoxically addressed in a promotional video made by Lego in collaboration with Andrés Ruzo, a National Geographic explorer. In the product endorsement clip, Ruzo explains that the Jungle Exploration theme is an opportunity for adventurous minds to engage with an environment that resembles the Amazon, a unique place that provides "clean air and water, and medicines for people all over the world." The ad hints at the legendary Inca lost city of Paititi as inspiration for the Lego exploration site, emphasizing that the true value of the jungle is not its gold, but its ecological value for the Earth.[17] Enthusiastically, Ruzo reminds viewers that the jungle is the home to local populations, his "Amazonian friends," and hence, not a lost site in time and space, adding that he uses "science to understand and teach others about this magical place." It remains nevertheless unclear what his position is about the extracted gems and golden statues, but the video, in general terms, encourages audiences (and potential toy buyers) to consider the importance of understanding the Amazon and its secrets. In the context of natural resources, this message is particularly pertinent in a time punctuated by a health and an environmental crisis, and when it truly matters that younger generations comprehend the gravity of the stakes. Overall, the positive and negative aspect of toys, through their visual and material dimensions, is their capacity to didactically disseminate worldviews and attitudes. As long as objects to play with keep shaping childhoods around the globe, they will most likely continue mirroring the dynamic between the natural world, cultural practices, and knowledge.

Epistemic Drawings

While toys retain a didactic value, in societies with rich written language traditions, children's books occupy a special place as instructional, educational, pedagogical, and knowledge transfer visual tools. Textbooks, in particular, are products of documentation processes envisioned to mediate content considered to be relevant for children, as they grow and become socially involved, and participants in specific epistemic communities. At a macro-level, "no science textbook, even the most basic one, is comprehensible in itself"[18] and neither is the case at a micro-level (basic textbooks). As much as a toy can operate as a reflection of ideas about health and nature, so do educational books, in formalized ways, communicate and circulate assumptions, beliefs, observations, and facts that each society considers worth teaching their future generations. Decisions on the intellectual architecture of textbooks respond to social, political, and economic stimuli. Illustrations, drawings, diagrams, photographs, and other visual formats, just as the texts, are the result of deliberation on behalf of the producers. A textbook provides plenty of cues about the worldviews of the community behind its creation and that includes presumptions and frames of reference about nature as a part of the scaffolding of medicinal practices or as an assemblage of phenomena and organisms that include animals, plants, and fruits.

A review of thirty-five textbooks from around the world reveals how different the topics of health and nature are addressed locally and how distinct the selection of images is in each case. The explanations accompanying the illustrations vary greatly according to the country in question. In a Hungarian visual dictionary, for example, it is not uncommon to find an explanation about the symbolism of flowers in religious terms. Young readers quickly not only learn that *liliom* (lilly) has a strong smell but also that it stands for purity.[19] Since the audiences are children, some conceptualizations pose challenges, such as the implicit occupancy of beds as prerequisites for a "hospital" to exist in a Kenyan textbook.[20] While in others, social prescriptions operate as filters to interpret and explain the natural world, as shown, for instance, by the sample sentence chosen for the word "natur" in Danish: "vi må ikke smide affald i nature" (we are not allowed to throw trash in nature).[21] Taxonomies differ considerably as well. In a Kyrgyz book, for example, the classification of animals includes pets, farm animals, animals from the woods, animals from the North, animals who live in "warm countries" (27), and some other animals (e.g., kangaroo).[22] In contrast, a Polish visual dictionary makes a distinction between pets, farm, and forest animals, animals *destined* to live in the zoo and those found in the grass.[23]

Textbooks to learn foreign languages also reveal interesting aspects of how the topics of health and nature are shown. In a Polish-English thematically divided illustrated dictionary, for instance, besides the basic vocabulary needed for situations classified under "Choroby i zdrowie" (Health and Illness), the author includes, presumably humorously, the sentence "mam alergię na szkołę" (I am allergic to school). The witty undertone is further confirmed by the complementary sentence, "Co jeszcze byloby dostatecznym pretekstem, żeby zostać w domu?" (What else would be a satisfying excuse to stay at home?).[24] Both sentences are accompanied by images of distressed men being either consoled or assisted by women, a nurse in the second case. Another comic connotation follows on with the inclusion of a hotel resort as part of the physical geography theme, and a final subsection of the book bearing the title "Wymarzone miejsce" (Dream Place). The glossary of terms needed to describe Dream Place include "żadnych obowiązków" (no duties), "żadnych rachunków" (no bills), "lodówka pełna zimnych napojów" (fridge full of cold drinks), and "piaszczysta plaza z palmami tuż obok" (sandy beach with palm trees at hand).[25]

Representations of health oscillate between cartoonish illustrations of happiness and technical, somehow clinical illustrations. In German *Mein buntes Deutsh-Bildwörterbuch* (2001), being healthy is represented by a child named Uwe whose height is being measured. A motive Larousse uses in all the translations distributed across the world. Estimating the right weight and height is also rendered as a marker of health and care for the body in the Greenlandic visual dictionary *Assiliartalaersugaq* (2001). In like manner, Burmese အမြင်အာရုံအဘိဓာန် (*My Big Book of Pictures*) includes one entry for "medicine," portrayed by the image of an open jar of colorful pills pouring out of it. Three images that coherently endorse a medicalized approach to the assessment of health. Validated by its use in formalized instructional settings, textbooks have been influential in strengthening, indoctrinating, normalizing, or favoring views, echoing often the dominant attitudes among members of society at the time of publication. Except for visual dictionaries from Indonesia, Laos, and Uzbekistan, the concept of traditional medicine is not included.

Images and drawings used to complement the written texts and to transfer and frame knowledge provide cues about prevalent ideologies behind their selection and elaboration. Even if the content of textbooks might at times prove to be problematic, they do not routinely face much resistance from either teachers, parents, or pupils, precisely because they are considered authoritative written sources of information. Educational materials reveal various aspects of the culture behind their conception as they diligently register social, cultural, and epistemic transformations, as they take place, in the communities that use them. A classic example is the stark contrast between modern-day Australian history books and Walter Murdoch's infamous paragraph, written at the beginning of the twentieth century and meant as an explanation about historiography:

> When people talk about the history of Australia they mean the history of the white people who have lived in Australia. There is a good reason why we should not stretch that term to make it include the story of the dark-skinned wandering tribes who hurled boomerangs and ate snakes in their native land long ago before the arrival of the first intruders from Europe. (1929, 9)

Indigeneity as a notion is present in many of the books, nonetheless, in the form of communities presented to live in close connection with nature and to be knowledgeable about intangible and supernatural forces. Native peoples are portrayed to practice forms of medicine that are in sync with a philosophy where ecological concerns reign and a sense of wisdom grounded in millennial traditions. A case in point is the treatment of the topic of Indigenous medicine in the Belgian children's book *Indianen*, a picturesque compendium on Indigenous communities published originally in German with the title *Expedition Wissen: Indianer* (2008) and authored by Rita Steininger. Even from the well-intentioned positionality of an educative book for children,

Indianen is rich in stereotypes that recirculate long-established assumptions about native peoples. The book endorses the tradition of framing Indigenous knowledge visually and discursively as one in stark contrast with knowledge systems presumed to distinguish Western societies, even if the notion of the West, as such, is in itself paradoxical and somehow incoherent.[26] The author seems to assess the distance between Indigenous and non-Indigenous knowledge(s) according to the role that technology is assumed to play in each of the cases, championing the assumption that Indigenous epistemologies and applied sciences are discordant terms. This is an assumption that has harmed the inclusion and participation of native societies in colonial and postcolonial settings. A trope that visual culture has adopted and reproduced ever since the first encounter between the New and Old World took place, and a by-product of a tapestry of preconpetions prevalent in Europe for centuries.[27] As a result, in the realm of Western art, canons of representation of native peoples, with some exceptions, consistently underpin othering discourses and tropes that, by extension, allegedly avouch a tendency to mock, undervalue, or alienate Indigenous knowledge systems. In the process, Native American healing traditions are customarily not depicted as formal types of medicine, above all, because they are considered incompatible with modernity.

Animated Reflections

The figure of the Indigenous or the so-perceived collectivity of non-modern peoples is therefore crucial to understanding traditions and processes of visual framing of medico-natural, medico-cultural, and medico-scientific spaces. Visual embodiments of the non-modern are in themselves encounters with representational counterimages of what constitutes hegemonic definitions of knowledge and science, particularly if they are wrapped in enchanting formats. Similar to textbooks, animation offers entry points into uncharted dimensions for young audiences, who allured by the seductiveness of the motion of sequential images enter the vortex of ideas engraved in the illustrations they so much enjoy.[28] From the early stages of animation, it became evident that, despite the enchantment and apparent simplicity of the format, it had a role to play in the construction of cultural and epistemic repertoires, as much as in the dissemination of attitudes and worldviews, and which included reflections and references about nature and health. Consuming and producing animation is a social practice infused with ideological connotations, at times, erroneously underestimated. And yet, it is worth remembering that the oldest animation feature film ever made *El Apostol/The Apostle* was a political satire produced by Quirino Cristiani in Argentina in 1917 to criticize then-president Hipólito Yrigoyen. Since its inception, moving images created from drawings have never ceased to be powerful visual tools to reach wide audiences and dispense influential messages.

Throughout the twentieth and twenty-first centuries, the landscape of animation has changed significantly in terms of production, and yet, it has retained its dominancy and visibility across the cultural scene at a national, regional, and global level. At present, mass media outlets in most countries of the world include in one way or another animation as part of the content targeted at children—as well as many adults. The malleability of the medium to adapt to specific local contexts has enhanced its internationalization and continuous evolution. Animation has gone through various stages, linearly marked by the advent of technology and particularly revolutionized by the introduction of computerized techniques. Furthermore, strengthened by the possibilities of Internet-based platforms and franchise-derived economic and distribution models, the realm of animation, as any other extension of cinema, has become a profitable amalgamation of art and commerce. Since its inception, cinematography has demonstrated its suitability as a didactic tool, nonetheless, because of its role as catalyzer of human emotions, enriching our understanding of the dynamic between images and audiences at a psychological and cognitive level.[29]

This is a fusion that illustratively materializes in contemporary reflections on many subjects, being one of them, the notion of biomedicine, or the lack thereof. There are examples in animated series of storylines in which the figure of the doctor or nurse is central, the hospital fulfills a key role as background to the narrative, a laboratory and its mysteries become a source of inspiration, or a pharmacy is a catalyzer for a series of events. Since exaggeration is a fundamental trait of the format, animated stories follow canons that playfully underline elements that make characters, locations, and situations recognizable at first sight. This applies to medicine-related themes, as much as it applies to the visual representation of nature. The physical world with all its encompassing elements, such as landscapes, animals, and plants, has unparallelly served as an influence for illustrators in their task of creating entrancing imagery. There are countless examples of animated zoomorphic characterizations of human societies, rituals, and traits. In like manner, picturesque anthropomorphic representations of the vegetative and mineral kingdoms as living beings, for example, with the capacity of speaking, convey a need to express how they are imagined and perceived. As any other art form, animation has made it possible for artists to transpose their sensitivities and anxieties onto optic illusions of intangible, abstract, or hard-to-grasp phenomena, such as rain, snow, thunders, or mist. Talking clouds, a prehistoric sable pondering about life, or a stubborn female oyster complicating matters for her diligent boss—a crab (e.g., *Glu Glú*, Chile, 2007)—are not just trivial entertainment outlets. Through animation, it is actually possible to visualize interpretations of nature as a trope and as a set of phenomena to which societies react on their own terms and according to their needs. Restoration of health is impendent to secure the continuation of life and animation registers this in many ways, ranging from the deployment of complex equipment to the use of magic. It is a genre where there are no demands of either accuracy or logic, and yet, many animated productions are repositories of stereotypical canons of representation.

As in the case of books, Indigenous epistemologies are the raw material for content in animation. Allusions to the wisdom of native peoples take many forms, but they seem to share in common two aspects worth mentioning. On the one hand, these narratives stimulate audiences to envision communities that have managed to remain outside knowledge regimes that involve the adoption of techniques, artifacts, and practices derived from artificial or artifactual approaches. On the other hand, animated storylines tend to approach Indigenous epistemic systems as the channelization of deep acquaintance with natural forces, apparently invisible to the untrained eye. In this sense, a reflection about the visuality of Indigenous knowledge unavoidably prompts a discussion of what knowing, doing science, and practicing medicine means, or how they are imagined and understood. Tacitly and recurrently, animated scenarios imply that a stethoscope is instrumental to a physician, as much as an immaterial force, cacophonic gestures, or magic powder are imperative to practice Indigenous medicine. A difference is made between learning how to cure and being endowed with the power of restoring health.

The trajectory of this old idea has taken many forms, but one recent example thereof is the characterization of natural remedies, science, technology, and progress in the French animated series *Nawak* (2021). Directed by Fabien Limousin and broadcasted by France 4 as televised and platform-based content, the 78 seven-minute episodes are conceived to target at five- to seven-year-old children. The series revolves around eponymous Nawak and his loyal friend Kawak—a pony that physiologically resembles a dog but behaviorally epitomizes a close friend to the young boy. The mutual dependency of Nawak and Kawak is key for the main character to deal with the consequences of his, often, poorly elaborated plans. Nawak's clumsiness, unluckiness, and messiness invariably result in a reaction on behalf of the short-tempered chief of the community or of the other members of the small society. In line with archetypical premises easily found in cartoons and comics about the Wild West, their skins are red-toned, wear feathers, and live in teepees on top of a large arid boulder in the middle of a densely forested corner of the globe. The scenario, storyline, and character building do not deviate much from European representations of native American lifestyles, which often include restyled elements taken from Hollywood characterizations. Specifically, according to Limousin, Nawak is inspired by *Yakari*, a popular Franco-Belgian comic book series first published in 1973 and widely adapted and translated to other formats and languages. Originally authored and drawn by two Swiss men—acclaimed comic writer Job (André Jobin) and illustrator Derib (Claude de Ribaupierre)—*Yakari* retains its place as one of the best-known Francophone comics. Besides the inexpertness of the main character, *Nawak* also differs from *Yakari* in the use of language. Except for undistinguishable guttural sounds and at times noises that superficially resemble actual sentences, in Nawak's world, communication is limited to exaggerated gestures, gesticulations, and screams. It is difficult not to make a connection between a long tradition of presenting Indigenous languages as background noise in cinema or as accidental hubbub in television with no coherent meaning whatsoever. On that account, it is also unavoidable to link the name of the series to the colloquialism *c'est nawak*, which stands in French for gibberish or nonsense. In the episodes that address health-related matters, the absence of spoken language is marked by rhythmic noises that resemble some form of spiritual chanting.

In the world of *Nawak*, the member of the community in charge of medicinal questions is a character whose name, status, or specific function remains undisclosed, but whose physical appearance and attire resemble visual representation of Native American Indigenous medicine men, African healers, curanderos, Siberian shamans, and wisemen. One might tend to assume it is a male figure, although his or her gender is another aspect that remains up for interpretation. Physically, the healer gives the impression of having been inspired by Ahtna medicine men capes captured in photographs in the twentieth century (figure 2.1). For the sake of this discussion, I will refer to this character as Magic Healer, due to the supernatural dimension of her/his curative and therapeutic techniques. They mostly revolve around dancing swiftly while moving arms and legs somehow choreographically for few moments. As a result, Magic Healer manages to create either a potion, a powder solution, or a flask that contains a cure to the problem at hand.

An example of this ability is shown in the episode entitled *Le Nez/The Nose*. What seems to be an idyllic apple gathering trip to the forest turns out the beginning of an eventful and quite strenuous day for the chief of the community. When trying to grasp the shiniest apple of a random tree in the forest, a competition ensues between the chief and a sly squirrel who also wants the apple for itself. The man-animal contest becomes a quest the chief is not willing to lose. Feeling defeated, after falling from the tree and bruised as a result of his encounter with the squirrel, he requests the presence of the Magic Healer at once. Having understood the gravity of the matter, the Magic Healer realizes he/she needs to create a potion that has the power to separate things apart. By virtue of the magic of his brisk movements and noises, the healer produces a flask with a green substance (figure 2.2).

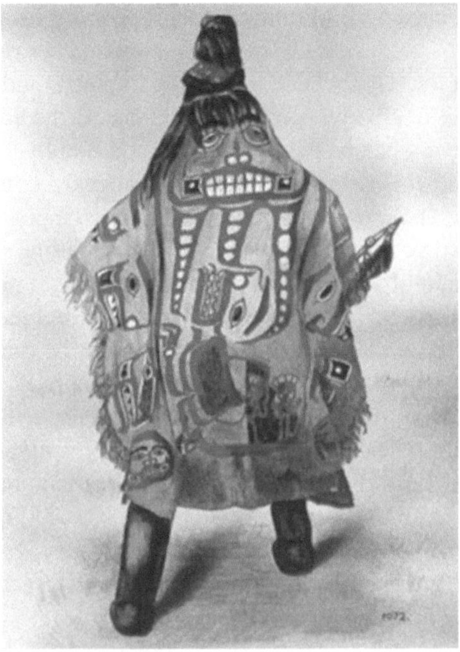

Figure 2.1 An Ahtna Indian Medicine Man of Alaska. *Source*: Colored photograph, ca. 1913. Wellcome Collection. Public Domain Mark.

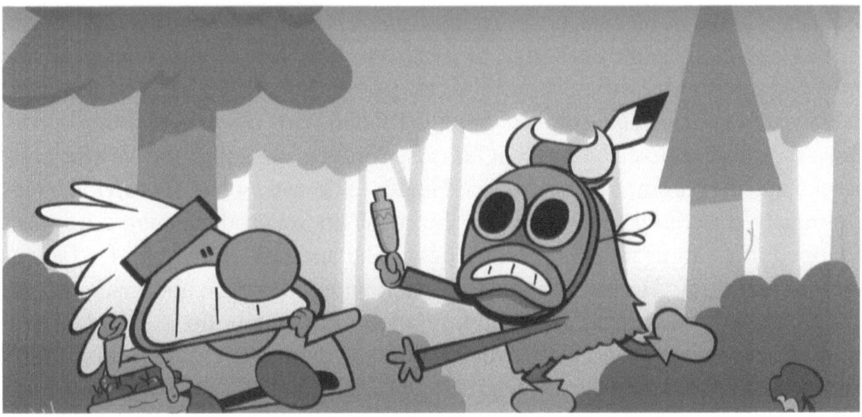

Figure 2.2 Screenshot from *Nawak* (2021).

A drop of which prompts the tree to release every single apple on the ground. However, things do not go as planned. In retaliation, the disappointed squirrel throws a half-eaten apple at the healer, propelling him to release the magic potion into the air. Accidently, part of the content of the flask ends up on the chief's nose, causing it to immediately drop from his face. Matters complicate even further. The flask with the magic potion gets tossed in the air again and finally lands on the chief's head, shattering in pieces and leaking the rest of the content of his face and body. As originally intended, the liquid prompts things to split apart, and every major piece of the chief's body gets dismembered—a scenario that, due to the nature of animation, appears comic and ingenious, rather than overtly graphic or grotesque. Nevertheless, it poses a conundrum for Nawak, who feels responsible to help the chief by putting together the pieces of his body in the right order although he does not seem to manage on his own.

Magic Healer offers to help by providing a detailed sketch with instructions and arrows that guide him on how to assemble each member in the right place. After trying many times with no result, Nawak finally manages to restore the chief back to his original form. There is nevertheless an issue that still demands attention. The nose is missing. Revengefully, the squirrel grasps it and escapes with it, forcing brave Nawak to chase the quick rodent across all the corners of the forest. Strangely, even if far away, the chief is able to trace and experience the trajectory of his nose. Water would leak from his nostril cavities, for instance, if his missing part was to accidentally fall into a river, or he would feel the pain of being stung by a poignant cactus if his nose was to be found stuck in a cacti shrub. Fortunately for the chief, at some point, thanks to the bravery and concerted efforts of Nawak, he manages to regain his missing part. Yet, not everything has been solved. The chief's nose is covered in the barbed bristles or spines, left by the cacti, and removing them causes the nasal structure to deflate entirely. Shocked by this unforeseen turn of events, Nawak uses glue to patch the hole left on the surface of the nose and eventually inflate it with an air pump. Too much air, nevertheless, overstretches the already highly damaged facial part, leading to a tragic end. Once the chief realizes he has lost his nose forever, the authoritative character breaks in tears, prompting the Magic Healer to devise a plan. Recurring to his previously described technique, he/she manages to produce magic powder, wrapped in a fabric pouch. A shiny new nose appears on the chief's face as soon as the Magic Healer sprinkles the yellow powder right above his mouth.

The episode closes in a celebratory mode but opens up a set of reflections about the representation of Indigenous medicine in visual culture easily summed up in two questions: First, is it productive not to dare imagining, even if it only happens fictitiously through infantile visualizations, that there might be more than one way of knowing and healing? And second, isn't it time to realize that nature and the natural world as concepts vary according to the pursuit of the epistemic system in question? There is perhaps no way to answer these questions, but the series of stamps reviewed in the next section indicate there is willingness to create pictorial idealizations of knowledge, nature, and health.

MEDICAL PHILATELY

Health is too present in human daily life, and its visual presence has permeated formats much less formalized and academicized, such as the philatelic world. The circulation of mail and the visuality of postage stamps attached to it have also served as illustrative vehicles to convey ideas about health and nature. Wilderness, flora, and fauna are recurring motives in the creation of pictorial emblems that embody the essence of the countries issuing them. In the process, the display of not only landscapes, endemic animals, and iconic plants, but also the politics and rhetoric of self-representation register the evolution of ideas about the natural world. In the last three decades, in particular, ecological awareness has logically permeated into the philatelical realm. Stamps on the topic of the environment and environment protection have included the image of a woman sweeping around her home (Burkina Faso, 1987), the visible roots under a tree (Mozambique, 1990), a reforested hill (Eritrea, 1997), a symbolic phytomorphic collage (North Macedonia, 2002), the Earth in flames (Thailand, 2008), a person picking up trash (Senegal, 2008), and the choice of a reusable bag instead of a plastic one (Malta, 2021). Logically, agriculture and crops have also inspired and informed representations of nature as site to be managed, superimposed, and superintended by humans. Often, these stamps suggestively imply that there is a telluric connection between nation-estate, cultures, ethnicities, and the ecosystems they inhabit. Today as much as in the past, traces of colonialism are also easily identified in philatelic compositions. An example thereof is the figure of a Somali girl harvesting papaya fruits (*Carica papaya*) shown in figure 2.3. An image designed by Corrado Mancioli (1904–1968) as part of an assignment commissioned by Officina Governativa Carte Valori (Rome) and issued in 1961.

Directly and indirectly, biodiversity and a connection between harvests and well-being is a theme in stamps. Philatelic venues have served to offer renderings of the contrasts between, for instance, apples from different regions and from all corners of the world (e.g., issued in Yemen, 1967; New Zealand, 1969; Algeria, 1978; Chile, 1989; Madagascar, 1992; South Africa, 1994; Pakistan, 1997; Wallis and Futuna, 2001; Poland, 2002; Tajikistan, 2005; Papua New Guinea, 2013; Luxembourg, 2015). Yet, the visuality of crops and fruits, as Kevles (2020) shows in the case of heirloom apples in the United States, is not only revealing or pertinent from an aesthetic viewpoint. Iconicity is part of pomological history, as much as government interests, economic enterprises, techno-scientific inventions, visual politics, and, indeed, ideologies about nature, health, and well-being. Circulation of images emerged or derived from commercial settings serves a purpose.[30] Taking a recent example, one can always wonder in which way the 900-CFA-franc

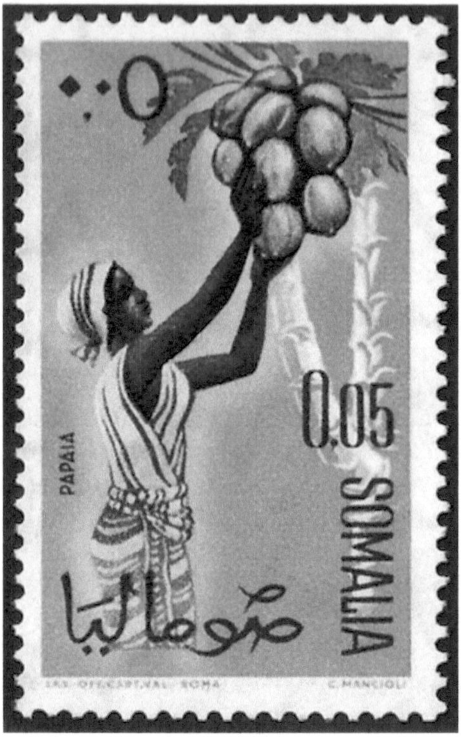

Figure 2.3 Stamp of the Somali Republic (Somalia), Issue "Crops," 1961. *Source*: Katarinaiv. Public Domain Mark.

stamp depicting an apple and released in March 2021 in the Central African Republic inscribes itself in the history of commodities, visual representation of crops, propaganda, advertisement, (neo)colonialism, and commerce.

As part of the vast repertoire of genres and media, stamps have retained for a long time their capacity to engender the atmospherics at the time of their production. This explains the diversity of themes. As noted by medical philatelists, topics such as history of medicine, health-related scenarios displayed in art, evolution of treatments, major breakthroughs, awareness campaigns, widespread diseases, prevention, vaccination campaigns, and promotion of health-enhancing practices and lifestyles constitute a subgenre in its own right.[31] Due to the importance of the theme, most countries have issued postage stamps related to the subject. Medical philately counts hundreds of pieces in their elaborated catalogs, almost 3,000, according to some estimates. The pictorial representation of health and nature is, for instance, central in the Health collection, issued in New Zealand in 1933 (figure 2.4) and as a subtheme in one of the Gandhi commemorative stamps released in 2020 in India.

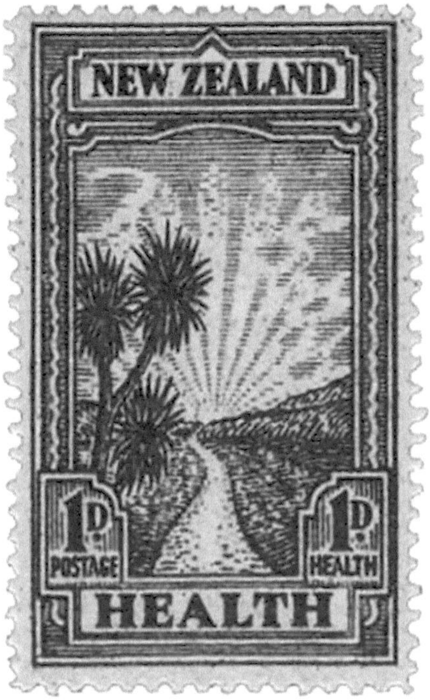

Figure 2.4 Public Health Stamp. New Zealand Postage Stamp, 1933. *Source*: Steve Strummer. Public Domain Mark.

Stamps mirror the heterogeneity of conceptualizations of health and medicinal therapies across cultures. In 2012, Romania issued, for instance, a collection of three stamps under the motto "Trăieşte sănătos" (Live healthy!) and featuring, among other garlic, tomatoes, nuts, berries, and honey. The motives underline the connection between specific types of food and prevention of diseases. Furthermore, the promotion of health includes awareness about practices that have proven to be harmful. Alertness about the damaging effects of smoking, for example, is a theme in stamps issued in Ethiopia (1980), Ivory Coast (1980), El Salvador (1983), Israel (1983), Yemen (1988), Slovenia (1993), Venezuela (1993), Brunei (1994), Dominica (2000), Tunisia (2005), Moldova (2011), South Africa (2015), Bosnia and Herzegovina (2019), and Syria (2020). Diseases such as cancer (Norway, 1953; Congo, 1966; Kuwait, 1970; Dominican Republic, 1974; Indonesia, 1987; Croatia, 1992; Turkey, 1997; Bolivia, 2001; Greenland, 2009; Curaçao, 2014; Liberia, 2016; Australia, 2020) and HIV (Vietnam, 1997; Colombia, 2000; Tuvalu, 2004; Ghana, 2006; Portugal, 2006; Sri Lanka, 2011; Sierra Leone, 2016; Togo, 2019) are the central leitmotif in stamps from all corners of the globe. The promptness and responsiveness of visual renderings of current affairs show in the collection of stamps that are currently (2021) registering the implications of Coronavirus (Chad, 2020; Guinea-Bissau, 2020; Guyana, 2020; Spain, 2020). Subsequently, the eventual vaccination for COVID-19 has also entered the philatelical domain (Zimbabwe, 2021), as part of a tradition of issuing stamps about the treatment and cure for diseases.

The philatelic articulation of therapeutic methods seems to mirror hierarchized distinctions between biomedicine and traditional medicine. Visually, the portrayals of pharmacological preparations (United States, 1972; Trinidad and Tobago, 1982; Norway, 1995; Spain, 2003), injections (Nigeria, 1968; Samoa, 1996; Angola, 2019), and pills (Afghanistan, 2004; Spain, 2008) differ from the depiction of traditional medicines (Sri Lanka, 2020). A commonality is that the focus lies on the epistemic aspect of dispensing precursors to treat illness. The visual representation of traditional medicine are predominantly images of raw seeds, leaves, roots, and fruits (Vietnam, 1993; Macau, 2003; Mozambique, 2005; Colombia, 2012). Another characterization features herbal remedies, either in the form of flowers (Bulgaria, 1981) or as preparations (Jamaica, 2005).[32] As in the case of other formats, stamps register health and nature as concepts deeply embedded in each culture. Visual depictions report on the idiosyncratic elements that define how each society relates to the cure and care of the body while capturing in images the sense of bioclusivity that inspires them.

NOTES

1. Pitarakis (2021).
2. Lbova (2021).
3. Jenkins (1998).
4. On femininities and masculinities, see Kimmel (2001), Philips (2001), and Pilling (2012).
5. Alexandratos (2017).
6. Farshtey (2013).
7. The description of the City Hospital set on Lego's official site reads: "Grab your stethoscope and head to the 60204 LEGO® City Hospital, where heroes are needed every day! This amazing set features a hospital building with reception area, kiosk and ambulance drop-off, vision testing room with eye chart, x-ray room with a light brick function, plus an operating/delivery room. It's also modular, so you can configure it in different ways. This cool set also includes an ambulance with opening back door and space for a stretcher, a helicopter with spinning rotors and storage box, and a separate buildable helipad. Includes 11 LEGO minifigures, plus skeleton and baby figures. Includes 11 LEGO® minifigures: 3 doctors, a hospital worker, 2 paramedics, mom, dad and 3 patients, plus skeleton and baby figures. Features a modular, 3-level hospital building with reception area, kiosk and ambulance drop-off, vision testing room with

eye chart, x-ray room with light brick function, plus an operating/delivery room and a helipad. Also includes an ambulance with opening back door and room for a stretcher, plus a helicopter with spinning rotors and storage box. Configure the hospital modules to create your own unique hospital design! Spin the rotors on the helicopter to transport needed medical supplies in the storage box. Lift the back of the ambulance to unload the minifigure patient on the stretcher. Flip the switch to trigger the light brick and take an x-ray. Accessory elements include a stretcher, stroller, flowers, head bandage, baby bottle, baby bed, rolling shelves, scissors, syringe, needle, 2 cupcakes and 3 bottles, plus a buildable wheelchair" (Lego Official Site, 2020).

8. An approach identified in Lego minifigures featuring other settings as well (Gonzalez Rodriguez, 2020).

9. For instance, through tangible objects and attributes about those objects (Hurtienne, Stößel, and Weber, 2009).

10. Peeren (2020) reminds us that Lego toys have the capacity of creating "immersive engagement" with scenarios that are paradoxically "reenactments of colonial and penal discipline" settings, such as the prisoner figurines that offer the possibility of *playing at* and *playing with* the idea of being in prison (6).

11. Sheina et al. (2017); Önder (2018).

12. Johnson (2014); Black, Tomlinson and Korobkova (2016); Gutwald (2017).

13. The snake charmer stereotype has a long history in popular culture (Gindhart, 2014; Hanson, 2014; Racy, 2016; Sharma, 2017).

14. On the issue of gender stereotypes, Lego has a dedicated section of its official website to present results from a study on the matter and a corporate statement: "Billund, October 11th: New research commissioned by the LEGO Group reveals that girls today feel increasingly confident to engage in all types of play and creative activities, but remain held back by society's ingrained gender stereotypes as they grow older. The study was carried out by the Geena Davis Institute in recognition of the UN's International Day of the Girl and to mark the launch of a new LEGO® campaign, 'Ready for Girls', which celebrates girls who rebuild the world through creative problem solving. The research, which surveyed nearly 7,000 parents and children aged 6–14 years old in China, Czech Republic, Japan, Poland, Russia, UK and USA highlights the need for society to rebuild perceptions, actions and words to support the creative empowerment of all children [. . .]. Our commitment: Ensuring more inclusive play and raising the debate around gender norms is critical, not just for girls but for any child. The LEGO Group knows that boys are also battling prejudice when it comes to creative play and playing with toys that are traditionally seen as being for the opposite sex. 71% of boys vs. 42% of girls say they worry about being made fun of if they play with a toy typically associated for the other gender. The company is committed to making LEGO play more inclusive and ensuring that children's creative ambitions—both now in the future—are not limited by gender stereotypes. We know there is work to do which is why from 2021, we will work closely with the Geena Davis Institute on Gender in Media and UNICEF to ensure LEGO products and marketing are accessible to all and free of gender bias and harmful stereotypes" (Lego Official Site, 2021).

15. Mbembe (2019).

16. Forgetting that there are also other ways of looking at the negotiations that underpin the production of science as Soto Laveaga (2009) insightfully demonstrates in the case of yam farmers in twentieth-century Mexico.

17. In her meticulous study about Paititi as a site, Roy (2017) notes that the mystical place can refer to "1) mythical tales, sometimes superimposed on the myth of Inkarrí, that place Paititi in a hidden town in the jungle, where the sovereign beheaded by the Spanish waits patiently for the moment to return and reestablish his power; 2) stories about 'ruins,' where Paititi is the name attributed to real archaeological remains: these stories have the particularity of mixing the legends related to the 'treasures' locked up in the town of Paititi and very specific geographic data that led to more than once to locate archaeological sites—Julian Tennant in 1958 in the Vilcabamba archaeological park, Herbert and Nicole Cartagena in 1979 in the Manu National Park; 3) testimonies that contain colonial historical sources, where Paititi is presented as a distant kingdom located in the jungle area west of the Andes, to which the Incas—Pachacutec, Tupa Yupanqui and Huayna Capac, if all the versions studied are considered—sent expeditions, and where some members of the elite took refuge upon the arrival of the Spanish" (107).

18. Schemmel (2012), 271.

19. Bánki (2010).

20. Waimitila (2009).

21. Jakobsen and Vissing (2011), 112.

22. Zhaychybekov (2012).

23. See Stadford (2015).

24. Interestingly, in Lang (2015), the Polish word "lekarstwa" is entered as the translation of "medicines" and "cures" in English and are portrayed as a blue and brown bottles next to each other. Since the words for tablets and pills are found listed somewhere else, the decision to include the term "cures" seems intentional, perhaps an attempt to recognize Polish folk medicine and remedies.

25. Lang (2015).

26. Appiah (2018).

27. Ouweneel (2018).

28. It matters how messages are diffused among children in media (Gross, 2002; Wells, 2008; Moyer-Gusé and Riddle, 2009; O'Shaughnessy and Stadler, 2010; Marsh, 2013), through animation (Björkqvist and Lagerspetz, 1985; Ginneken, 2007; Artz, 2015; Driscoll, 2011; Batkin, 2018), through videogames (Dovev and Kennedy, 2007; Penix-Tadsen, 2013), and through literary sources (Diaz Soto, 2000; Stephens, 2002; Bradford, 2007).

29. Laukötter (2016).

30. Visual representations of fruit, as Klein (2020) demonstrates, figuratively can also be reflections on the politics of food and the intersection between art, technology, imperialism, and racism.

31. Bishop and Murdoch Matheson (1948); Kler (1969).

32. Part of the commemorative issue of the 200th anniversary of Mary Seacole's birth.

Part II

SHAPES OF NATURE

Chapter 3

Barcoded Pharmacopeias

Morphologically, nature acquires various shapes and silhouettes as it travels through networks created to harness its medicinal properties in one way or another. The trajectory of plants and herbs perceived to enhance human health, and their users, undergoes various stages, from collection to preparation and distribution. In the process, nature mutates, adapts, and adjusts to the spaces where it plays different roles at different moments. The inherent need to retain and restore health has translated into the creation of habits of consumption that are equally cultural, epistemic, transactional, environmental, and political. Before arriving to the shelf of a store, plant-based medicines, specially those from so-perceived exotic locations, or promoted as borrowings from ancient epistemic systems, are anticipated by the circulation of the idea that nature heals, is available for sale, can be harnessed for one's benefit, has no implications for the future of fragile ecosystems, and is universal property. Colorful small bags, picturesque minimalist containers, stylishly designed flasks, or appealing jars embody the various visual presentation of nature as a cure, remedy, preventive treatment, or health enhancer. Overabundance of consumables for the care and cure of the body in the twenty-first century is best articulated by their overrepresentation in digital ecosystems and their global circulation—a process in which language plays a crucial role.

CIRCULATION OF ENDEMICNESS

SKU: 037410 is one of the codes used to label Purasana Moringa© in some of the many stores where the product is sold across Western Europe. According to the description, it is a bag of raw powder produced by minimally processing the leaves of the *Moringa Oleifera* tree, also simply known as moringa or ben oil tree.[1] Stirring three teaspoons of the powder in any drink, such as fruit juice, is one of the many ways of ingesting the nutritious properties of the plant, according to the enclosed recommendations. The details in the package or in the promotional material state that the plant "staat bekend" (is known) for its medicinal properties. The vagueness of this description is paradoxically opposite to the specificity of moringa's stock-keeping unit (SKU) codes. SKU codes are scannable references that label and track the movement of units sold in a retail store. All moringa-derived products have different scannable bar codes, of course, even if the main component is the same. The singularity of the original plant is traversed by the plurality of needs of markets designed to quench the thirst of various types of users and their appetite for various versions of moringa, retaining its original qualities. The erectness of the tree resembles the verticality of bars that make up a code readable only by numeric interfaces connected to digital networks that classify, categorize, and tally how plant-based merchandise sells and how much of it. Either the leaves or parts of the bark and branches are marketed according to a hierarchy where rawness, purity, and additional ingredients define the price and greenness of the product. These codes not only follow the path of consumables from the stock room to the shelves and from the shelves to the cashier's hands, but they also follow the customer as they get printed on a receipt that the salesperson hopes not to see again, for instance, in case the client decides to bring the item back or ask for compensation.

Little information is shared by stores selling natural products about the number of customers demanding a reimbursement, claiming that the natural medicines fail to meet their expectations. The list of medicinal properties on the package conveys a sense of ambiguity and impreciseness, but expressions such as "superfood," "raw healthy," "vegan immunity," and "green power" soon dissipate (or are expected to dissipate) any doubt. Natural products and those on a gray area between food, medicines, remedies, supplements, and nutraceuticals (food that provides medical or health benefits) are sold in bags that seal not only their content but also the secrets of the origins, collection, processing methods, and the impact of consuming them at a large scale. Moringa, like other hundreds of plants, constitutes the basis of a market underpinned by the materialization of naturality in consumables widely available to anyone as food and nutraceuticals. Many studies have been conducted on *Moringa oleifera* with diverse results.[2] They do not always back up the claims on the labels, but that fact does not necessarily obstruct their circulation or affect their marketing strategies. The labels on the products furnish information about the purported therapeutical use of their natural precursors and function as simplified points of references. In that sense, the packages and promotion material resemble fragmented abstractions of modern-day barcoded pharmacopeias.

Images and texts on packages of plant-based health and wellness consumables focus, above all, on implying that the contents are direct extractions from nature. In the circulation of images of health-restoring, -enhancing, and -improving natural precursors, the notions of endemicness and naturality play a central role. I argue that endemicness, understood as the quality of occurring naturally and being prevalent in a particular place, is a two-pronged concept. On the one hand, it refers to the native origin of the plant in question and, on the other, to the ancestry of the epistemic system that underpins the purported knowledge about its medicinal properties. Naturality and endemicness function to various extents, consistently, although not coherently as a visual and semiotic strategy to convey a sense of trust. Commonly held assumptions about traditional epistemic systems and healing practices validate any statement. Bivins (2007) observes that well-recognized distinction separates standardized and non-standardized operationalization of therapeutic practices. Self-medication is commonplace in informal spaces where phytomedicinal formulas and ethnobotanical nutraceuticals are free to circulate.[3] Their visual and virtual presence denote the lax regulations surrounding products easily labeled as natural, often considered extensions of alternative medicine, and, hence, not subject to strict regulations. Moringa is sold across the European Union as superfood, "superleaf," gut health product, vegan snack, health-promoting powder (figure 3.1), and the basis for over 50 types of cosmetics. It can be eaten and applied externally, and there does not seem to be any limit to its efficacy or versality. Part of the introductory text about moringa includes references to its reputation as a medicinal plant in Asia. This somehow brings to mind the tendency to associate aboriginal, native, and Indigenous cosmologies with methods to harness the presumed illimited faculty of nature to restore health. Brown (2016) asserts that this connection is furthermore underlined by the figure of Mother Earth, oral tradition, spirituality, and phytotherapies. On that account, medicines with dubious scientific properties can be understood as the materialization of complex processes where culture is mediated for economic purposes.[4] In that sense, acculturation and inurement of endemicness as a trait facilitates the process by which any exotic plant can potentially become the basis for a purported nutraceutical.

The routine, mundane, and yet indispensable role food plays in daily life explains not only the emotional and sensorial relation humans have with edibles but also the importance of branding in the creation of products that seduce and convince consumers. Food has been approached from a historical and political standpoint, in connection with gender, as an identity marker linked to social interaction and, in general, as a part of material culture intrinsically linked to daily rituals and practices.[5] The aesthetic component

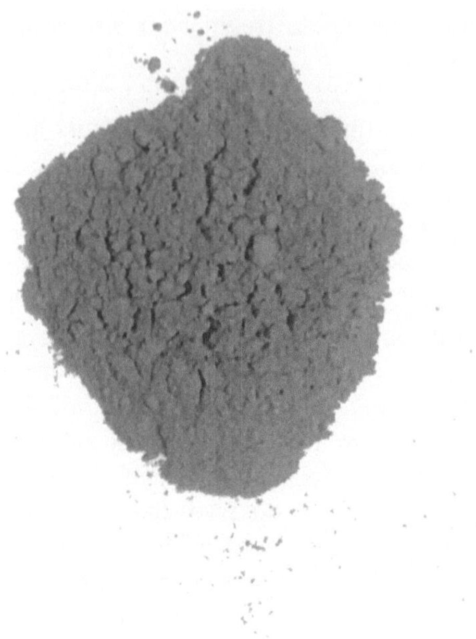

Figure 3.1 Moringa-Based (*Moringa oleifera*) powder. *Source*: Photo by author.

of food and its impact, in this case, on shoppers, is as important as the values that it elicits. Values, I suggest, are filtered through their own bioclusivity interdependencies. Ideas about the content of food, the technology used in its production, its origin, and the various meanings attached to the various types of consumable goods explain why framing food products visually requires positioning these items as not only gastronomical and palatable but also ideological and cultural artifacts. Fruits, seeds, and grains that are framed and branded as ancestral, native, and hence natural, powerful, authentic, and pure ultimately make references to notions and ideas commonly held about Indigenous lifestyles now, and especially Indigenous eating practices imagined to have been the norm before colonization took place. An approach that resembles Schaffer's (2009) discussion on the linkage between presumed scientific sophistication and extinct ancient civilizations.

The visuality of endemicness is linked to cognitive and mnemonic processes intrinsically linked to cultural background, similar to the processes linked to the notion of indigeneity.[6] Preconceptions about a specific social group and ethnicity or a specific identity, even if it is informed by imagination, rather than facts, materialize in preconceived ideas linked to a set of characteristics that operate at various levels.[7] Along this line, Knight (2018) has shown that there is a tendency to idealize and contextualize indigeneity in terms of food production and technologies. As it seems, consumable goods that are not considered to be modern or Western are easily associated with claims about health-enhancing properties.[8] More than ever before, in the last decades, "The marketing of native foods reflects and reinforces the notion that indigeneity is a category that exists outside of the cultural."[9] To some degree, it becomes a notion easily applicable, attachable, malleable, and flexible enough to decorate, complement, enhance, and legitimize the promotion of food that elicits certain values among its possible consumers (e.g., authenticity, purity, greenness, freshness, and healthiness).

An imagined origin is then equated to assumptions and sensitivities closely related to concerns about its locative dimension and origin. Imaginaries (defined by our own bioclusivity) about food appear to apply to preconceptions, expectations, and anxieties about specific geographical places. Assumptions regarding the landscapes where these products grow and are manufactured contribute to their positioning within specific foodscapes.[10] Visually, Indigenous cultures, ornaments, languages, and settings (landscapes) become referents that legitimize and enhance the connection between ancestry, tradition, and perceived naturality and endemicness. The aesthetic and visual references deployed in the promotion of nutraceuticals cannot be underestimated. Nonetheless because the visibility and credibility of the plants and herbs in question depend on the associations potential patients/consumers make between the provenience and medicinal efficacy of the raw materials. A "scientific-non-scientific continuum" underlines the centrality of the rhetoric,[11] graphic, and symbolic aspects of the naturality-endemicness dyad in the context of nutraceuticals. The capacity of the plants to be transformed into marketable outputs is then correlated with preconceptions and a set of beliefs held by the potential buyers, mostly in industrialized societies. An aspect that denotes the sense of bioclusivity in nations that entwine *real* nature with tropes about exoticism, foreignness, and tropicality. In the context of the relation between societies, their ecosystems, and healthscapes, it remains equally important to understand how these embodiments of the natural world unfold and affect countries where raw materials are produced.

Visual Naturality and Indigeneity

Reviewing the advertisement posts of 35 companies from 6 Latin American countries dedicated to the production of natural food medicines and (phytopharmaceutical) nutraceuticals, the emerging pattern is the connection producers make between visual stimuli, nature, indigeneity, and origin of the plant/herb in question. Imaginaries and ideas about the power of medicinal herbs are closely linked to expectations (52%), preconceptions (34%) and anxieties (16%) about specific geographical places. Ideas about the landscapes where the plants grow and their natural state contribute to their sense of legitimization. The corpus of selected posts (N = 600) on Facebook confirms the connection phytomedicinal companies make between terms such as "native," "indigenous," "ancestral" (22%), and "concepts" such as "effective" (27%), "properties," and most commonly "natural" (51%). The endemicness/naturality dyad is tactically, but tacitly, used to promote and visually frame "powerful" medicines, complementary diet therapies, or alternative comestible healing practices. Products developed within an ethnobotanical approach deploy specific visual strategies and aesthetic codes in the creation of promotional campaigns. By documenting the responses and reactions of consumers of the products to the promotional material (i.e., packages and advertisements) used by the various phytopharmaceutical companies, it was possible to draw commonalities and patterns.

Rare plants, herbs, fruits, and trees are common references in illustrations and moving images that serve to promote "natural" products. Yet, a commonality across the spectrum of phytopharmaceutical products reviewed is the absence of factual information about the properties, effectiveness, and processes of production. Visual codes and cues are strategically deployed to insinuate that natural/Indigenous/ancestral methods of production, preparation, and consumption are free from the damaging effects of Western, less effective medicinal approaches. The encoding mechanism of the messages works as both consumers and producers make connections between the contents of the products, Indigenous knowledge, and health-promoting properties, specially supported by the notion that these herbs are part of century-old traditions. According to the reaction of consumers to digital spaces, lack of trust, anxieties, and concerns about contemporary pharmaceutical technologies explain the rejection some of them show to traditional medicine. The companies were selected based on their digital footprint, active use of social media platforms, number of followers, and visibility.

Throughout Latin America, it was possible to distinguish four strata: Andean Region (Inca Civilization), Mexican Region (Aztec and Maya Civilizations), Amazon Region (various "tribes"), and Unnamed Indigenous Landscapes, a series of locations allegedly, imaginatively, and inspirationally related to unnamed extinct Indigenous civilizations. Central to the subsequent discussion is to review how food technologies are promoted using as referent widespread assumptions held about pre-Columbian civilizations, similar to processes observed in Australia[12] and New Zealand[13] regarding imaginaries about precolonial food practices. In most cases, the marketing strategies indexically imply that products engender the epistemic legacy and biocultural heritage that characterize specific geographical places. By documenting the reactions of consumers to the advertisement and promotional material used by the various food companies, it was possible to make inferences about the way in which visual framing actually operates among the aiming audiences. In total, 35 digital promotional episodes were documented, one from each of the companies being analyzed. By episode, I refer to the actual posting of an image, the reaction of consumers, the interaction between consumers and producers, and the discussion between consumers.

Without exception, visual framing strategies of endemic products are linked to specific geographies and historical references about pre-Columbian agricultural knowledge. Claims about growing and harvesting traditions are added to images of raw materials lying on pieces of soil, often still covered in mud, piled up in a disorganized fashion, exposed to the sun, outside, or in the vicinity of green fields where human presence is imperceptible. Inclusion of pictures of the crops where the products allegedly grow and images of the finalized item ready for consumption is a common strategy. In the case of products destined for local markets, artisanal, poorly elaborated pseudo-infographics are deployed as part of the introductory phase of a new product. Complementary explanations, advice, and a list of health-enhancing properties in fonts written in earthy colors apparently encourage consumers to consider the innovative aspects of the product. At the same time, the Indigenous origin, sense of ancestry, and homage to traditions induced by visual references such as drawings, use of Indigenous languages, emblems, and symbols prompt viewers to consider these products are directly connected with the figure of the Indigenous. Indigenous emblems include drawn faces of natives wearing pre-Columbian attires, animals decorated with items commonly assumed to be ancient, patterns used in traditional clothing still worn by self-identified Indigenous communities, and images of landmarks closely related to precolonial times.

Across the Andean region, images and references to the mountains, old ruins built by Inca civilization (i.e., Machu Picchu), are comparable to the use of Maya ruins in the promotion of consumables grown in the Yucatan Peninsula in Mexico. In both cases, members of modern Indigenous communities wearing traditional clothes are also present(ed) in promotional visuals. Brazilian companies frame their food products mostly by appealing to the cluster of ideas that ascribe notions such as "mystery," "powerful," "Mother Earth," and "wisdom" to the Amazon Basin. Images of tropical landscapes covered by dense vegetation dominated by exotic trees and covered by unruly, massive forests are widely used to promote products fruits, seeds, and herbs. Drawings of naked Indigenous peoples wearing feathers, decorative facial and body paintings, and barefoot seem to represent a state of mind and being that is unrelated to industrialized, civilized, and standardized urban lifestyles. The use of Indigenous languages is widespread among the companies self-promoting themselves as producers of natural food products. With few exceptions, their names are in Amerindian languages; follow the spelling rules of languages such as Quechua, Mayan, or Tupi; and are distinguishably transformed into logos that convey the notion of simplicity, rurality, exoticism, and primitivism. The concept of superfood (i.e., Spanish/Portuguese *superalimento*) is directly linked to the peculiar, unrivaled properties of those fruits, seeds, vegetables, and grains grown in specific places and preserved by ancient civilizations that managed to stay healthy for centuries.

Pictorially, the images used to promote superfoods appeal to widespread ideas and myths about "lost" healthy practices and diets embedded in the knowledge of pre-Columbian societies. The captions and texts that accompany the images are often warnings about the importance of turning away from "modern," ineffective eating patterns. Concerns about overweight, health issues, and environmental problems are also used as a rationale for the need to include this series of products in modern diets. With few exceptions (N = 4), consumers agree with the claims made by the companies promoting the products. In fact, many display signs of agreement and (overinflated) praise (N = 304). Over 100 consumers react by providing information about additional properties not mentioned in the ads, while others simply thank for the information being provided and hope there are more similar products in the making (N = 88). As a trend, once the advertisement ads are posted on Facebook, Instagram, and YouTube, comments often surround around elevating the health-enhancing qualities of the product and its benefits. From this angle, it is possible to conclude that digital platforms serve as didactic and disseminating tools to share (uncorroborated) health-related information.

In many cases, the figure of the Indigenous almost extinct *Other* and her/his lifestyle are framed in the context of survival, rarity, and extraordinariness. The notion of superfood is central in the creation of products that are legitimized by the belief that they are comparatively much healthier, purer, more wholesome, and more nutritious than other food products. Indigenous origin or connections to native communities serve mostly an ideological purpose. Visual elements that operate as references to millennial societies imply the products are safe, come directly from nature, and are consumed before "modern" times. As Craw (2008) observes the need to look for new diet models outside more "standard" food technologies explain, among other reasons, the emergence of nutritional primitivism. The branding strategies and visual framing tactics deployed in the promotion of Indigenous-inspired food products are based on the assumption that those who are in harmony with Mother Earth and know her best possess knowledge(s) the rest of us don't. The use of plants, lush landscapes, ruins, flowers, rudimentary-looking fonts, and tribal decorations all contribute to creating a sense of earthiness. Indigenous legends provide contextual references that metaphorically contribute to creating a sense of historicity while strengthening the notion of ancestry, heritage, and tradition. The Argentinean agricultural cooperative Viva el Monte, for instance, uses the image of Zapam Zucum to allude to the Indigenous deity that jealously protects nature and, in specific, the prosopis tree (*algorrobo* in Spanish) (*Prosopis algarrobilla*), often associated with the European/Middle Eastern carob tree (*Ceratona siliqua*).

Similarly, languages are used to secure that the visual elements are complemented with a phonetic, sounded equivalent that enhances the difference between these brands and other European-sounded names. This confirms the need to take distance from Western technologies, lifestyles, means and methods of production, and food practices. Wipala Healthy Snacks from Ecuador, for example, explain in their promotional ads that *wipala* means flag in Quechua and that the seven-colored flag (i.e., their logo) symbolizes Andean culture, philosophy, and solidarity among people.

Concerns about poor diets that lead to overweight and health issues increase the popularity of food products that are credited to possess unrivaled health-enhancing properties such as sugar-free, organic, and fit with vegan, vegetarian, and gluten-free diets. Although there are no images of exposed torsos or highly sportive models, the image of green landscapes seems to convey the notion that "natural" food products could never be fattening or cause any harm. All along, associations with simplicity are maintained and iconically supported by images where unruly nature dominates.

Discussion patterns elicited in the recollection of 600 digital entries posted by consumers on social media platforms show they recognize the claims made by the food producers. The fact that they add new properties to those already mentioned in the advertisements indicates they had previous assumptions about the product before they saw the actual image. A close analysis of the comments made by the consumers leads to conclude that the images visually embody preconceived ideas about the power of Mother Nature and the knowledge of Indigenous communities surrounding certain types of fruits, herbs, and vegetables. Prices are important topics of conversation in the thread of messages that follow a picture used for promotional purposes of popular items (e.g., specific types of quinoa or rare combinations of local and imported goods). For many, it is important to know how much these products cost and to make statements about the benefits of eating "local" and "ancestral," as opposed to "modern," not only from a health perspective but also from a financial viewpoint.

Ironically though, many of the companies' primary markets are in the United States, Europe, and Asia.[14] Superfoods and nutraceuticals are visually branded as Indigenous-related consumables and are widely sold outside Latin America, using as main premise, precisely their exotic origin. Food packaging of those products destined for foreign markets is mostly attuned to notions of cosmopolitanism and primitivism. Images of exotic settings, references to awe-inspiring rites, and alluring decorations are used to fabricate the idea that native communities are somehow connected to the product in question. The main difference between exported goods and those consumed globally is that the former are framed around communities living in the geographical space where the product grows, whereas in the latter case, the references allude to extinct civilizations. Rare plants, herbs, fruits, and trees are common references in illustrations, impressions, and moving images that serve to promote nutraceuticals. Yet, a commonality among this category of goods is the absence of factual information about their nutritional content. Visual cues are strategically deployed to insinuate that Indigenous/ancestral methods of production, preparation, and consumption are free from the damaging effects of "modern" industrialized agricultural approaches. These images encourage viewers to consume what they suggest is pesticide-free ancestral legacy. Some of the food items promoted by companies specialized in organic products offer better prices than comparable consumables believed to have a less good impact on human health. According to the reaction of consumers to digital spaces, anxieties, and concerns about contemporary food technologies explain the rejection some of them show to notions of massification, overproduction, and recentness. A link between the products in question and *unpolluted* native communities allegedly legitimize claims about their purity, freshness, healthiness, effectiveness, and wholesomeness. All along, visual and textual references to telluric knowledge(s) are used to legitimize the products in question, both in the abovementioned cases and the infographics discussed in the next section.

INFOGRAPHICS

Infographics are virtual-visual surfaces designed to present information, following composition canons that render them convincing and educational, for instance, on how healthy spirulina (*Arthrospira platensis*, *Arthrospira fusiformis*, and *Arthrospira maxima*) is. From a functional perspective, they contribute, in principle, to mediate summarized pieces of data, accompanied by explanatory images. Since health communication intrinsically depends on mechanisms that mediate knowledge, in the twenty-first century, the use of health-oriented infographics has increased. At present, they freely circulate across social media spaces, search engines, print media, and advertisements. Credibility, veracity, and framing of facts in visual culture remain an issue.[15] Specially when uncorroborated and unsubstantiated information is presented as evidence-based findings. Unavoidably, the content of the visualizations risks being steered purely by commercial reasons, exposing audiences to unsupported claims, or contradicting recognized protocols.[16] On this account, there are three aspects to consider. In the first place, the notion of efficacy becomes questionable in settings where verifiability is not guaranteed. In the second place, infographics allocate spaces to present innovations, as much as to recognize less prominent bodies of knowledge, which has advantages and disadvantages, as in the case of herbal medicines.[17] The third aspect is that these visualizations can be seen as democratic attempts to popularize dissemination channels by debunking and challenging the formal nature of academic externalizations. After all, through semiotic and hermeneutic mechanisms, infographics resemble pictorial communication formats used by scientists. The question remains how this is having an impact on the general approach to knowledge dissemination and what this could mean for, for example, scientific communities and their interaction with larger societies. Another side of this reflection is how visualizations become evidence of often-overlooked information and knowledge or the worldviews of forgotten segments of society. Additions in epistemic systems and cultural repertoires do not always follow conversations at a societal level on how to relate to new forms of knowledge (e.g., spirulina-based snacks).[18] In this space between communication and consumption, I suggest, infographics emerge as visual surfaces that rely on their pictographness (merged images with language) to appear informative and useful.

Infographics offer new possibilities to visually deliver a message,[19] and as the subsequent semiotic analysis of 22 spirulina-related visualizations shows, communicative approaches differ. In some cases, the blue-green cyanobacterium is simply commercialized as an excellent supplement in "smoothies." In others, the claims include suggestions that spirulina can "reduce" cancer and "in some cases, heal it."[20]

Thematically, in 10 cases, medicinal benefits receive more attention than an explanation of spirulina's biological composition or origin. In 12 infographics, the main topic is taxonomically compartmentalized medicinal properties. In seven cases, this is done following anatomical considerations, and in five cases, according to the most common ailments potential consumers have (e.g., lack of energy). Other subthemes, except in three cases, are spirulina's texture, presentation, optimal recommended consumption mode, and advised doses. References to biomolecules (22), specific organs (21), and envisioned results upon (regular/daily) consumption (17) confirm attempts to contextualize the message in biomedical terms. The use of icons (21), drawings (18), and illustrations (16) also suggest the authors deploy recognizable semiotic codes. One example includes the use of the breast cancer and HIV silk ribbons, without mentioning either disease. In the sentences where the main subject are specific diseases (themes), the most common rheme is the externalization of improved conditions. In the case of "digestion problems," consumption of spirulina would lead to "improved metabolism."

From a semiotic-linguistic perspective, the promotion of *Arthrospira* is specially interesting, I argue, because it denotes the ways in which language is instrumental in externalizing ideas about the nature-knowledge-health triad. Bearing in mind that epistemic transmission is the main function of infographics,[21] they rely on visual, as much as on pragmatic, lexical, and semantical codes. At a semantic level, three main fields are salient in the corpus, best epitomized through the verbs "increasing," "decreasing/lowering," and "helping." In all three cases, the pairing subfields are specific health conditions, symptoms, lifestyle impediments, possible risks, and mental/cognitive complaints. At a pragmatic level, indirect visual-linguistic allusions are made to gender-related concerns (e.g., menstruation cramps), environmental concerns (e.g.,"heavy metals detoxication"), and general well-being (e.g., happiness).

As for the lexical clusters, ditransitive and conative verbs are identified in 21 infographics. This is an important realization as it suggests that most of the spirulina visualizations adopt interactional patterns that resemble a conversation between a physician and a patient. In stark contrast with academic- or institutionalized research-based information dissemination patterns, the tone is more direct(ive). Caused motion (nine) and resultative (four) verbs are also found, but less so. A logical explanation for the presence of instructional clauses is the general functionality of (commercial) health-promoting visualization: engagement and endorsement. Examples of synonymy and meronymy involving medical vocabulary furthermore confirm that infographics are not intended to avoid associations with scientific information formats. On the contrary, spirulina is presented as an alternative to pharmacological preparations precisely through pharmaceutical-inspired visual iconicity and linguistic strategies. In the context of the discussion about the visuality of efficacy, images seem to be contextualized through language on three levels.

On one level, language is deployed functionally as a channel to convey a message about the therapeutic or healing qualities and properties of a precursor, practice, or object. The content of the texts accompanying the images is then usually descriptive, exhortative, hortative, homiletic, didactic, and instructive (i.e., advice about doses). The images and the captions depend on each other. On the second level, language moderates the message to suggest associations with an authoritative source of knowledge, particularly through biomedical and technical jargon (e.g., phycocyanin). In this case, linguistic strategies resemble the use of images. They mark visually the presence of references audiences recognize or think they do. The complexity of certain terms might prompt potential *readers* to turn into *viewers*. Instead of reading, for instance, names of complex molecules, they "view" them.[22] The word "carotenoids," in a spirulina-related infographic, I suggest, might be one of them. On the third level, I posit that infographics, as many newer formats, are intrinsically related to the twenty-first-century virtual turn by-products/-practices that merge language and images (pictographness). In that sense, infographics operate, on the one hand, as visual surfaces that present summarized information. But on the other hand, they are also visualizations that rely on the present-day preference for swiftness and speediness to convey a message embedded in an image intended to be seen but not necessarily fully understood. Since infographics convey data, even if the information is unsubstantiated, they fulfil nevertheless an epistemic function. Thus, they are a sample of epistemic-semiotic approaches through which the concept of medicinal efficacy is (mis)communicated. From that perspective, and bearing in mind the vast continuum between science and traditional knowledge in the context of therapeutic practices, language plays a *visual* role. This visuality, it seems, depends at all times on how images, texts, and their combination manifest the bioclusivity codes viewers/readers understand, recognize, and to which they relate.

NOTES

1. *Moringa oleifera* is also known as West Indian ben tree, horseradish tree, and drumstick tree.
2. See Joung et al. (2017); Sahai et al. (2017); Oleg et al. (2018); Kou et al. (2018); Matic et al. (2018); Nurdin et al. (2018); Das et al. (2019); Hasam et al. (2019); Okorie (2019); Biswas (2020); Meireles et al. (2020); Nova et al. (2020); Owens III et al.; Hedhili (2021); Mohanty et al. (2021); Zahidul et al. (2021).
3. In general, protocols for the production and commercialization of herbal medicines lack standardization (Kunle, Egharevba and Ahmadu, 2012).
4. Banerjee (2002) explores this point in the context of the commercialization of ayurveda.
5. Ferguson (2004); Counihan (2009); Kahn (1998); Gewertz (2010); Wilk (2007); Mintz and Du Bois (2002).
6. Ouweneel (2018).
7. See Leerssen (2007) on the concept of ethnotypes.
8. Loyer and Knight (2018).
9. Craw, 2008, 55.
10. Fraser (2017) observes that food systems are as much systems of oppression as they are systems of resistance.
11. Keshet (2009).
12. Knight (2008).
13. Craw (2008).
14. Peña-Lévano, Adams, and Burney (2020).
15. Richter et al. (2009); Mena (2021).

16. Elvin-Lewis (2001); Bent (2008).

17. Goldman (2001); Crawford and Leventis (2005); Valerio (2005).

18. Martucelli (2016).

19. Cairo (2012); Lankow et al. (2012); Otten et al. (2015).

20. Evidence of spirulina's effect on human health is inconclusive, but no study has convincingly shown it cures cancer. Studies about its possible applicability in cases of diabetes (Mehdinezhad et al., 2021), cardiovascular diseases (Sutelman et al., 2020), and antithrombotic properties (Koukouraki et al., 2020).

21. Pflaeging and Stöckl (2021).

22. On a conceptual level, this notion resembles Biagioli's (1990) discussion on the ways in which incommensurability and other interactional strategies relate to each other.

Chapter 4

Gendered Epistemic Artifacts

Visual representation has since antiquity registered the use of cosmetics as integral elements of rituals and gendered social practices that, beyond their ornamental connotations, have also signaled attempts to improve users' physical appearance, harmony, equilibrium, status, and health.[1] As previously discussed, culturally, across centuries, civilizations, and artistic canons, being well has materialized in renderings that associate the absence of disease with the presence of beauty, perfection, attractiveness, and good physical condition. There is a tendency to obviate the distinction between aesthetics and health, and how these unfold within each society's bioclusivity. For logical reasons, good health evokes notions of prettiness and appeal, diametrically opposite to the traits routinely equated with illness, or at least, absence of health. Looking well and appearing aesthetically pleasant matter and retain a social value.

Commercialization and mediatization of beauty and health come hand in hand, for instance, in the form of elective/voluntary plastic surgery, cosmetic dentistry, and rejuvenation treatments[2] although attempts to improve one's appearance most commonly involve engaging in home-based routines than in extensive undertakings. To various degrees, cosmetics hold a place in each culture, securing a high demand for items consumed and worn by many on a daily basis, not surprisingly, securing approximately 532 billion dollars in revenues in 2019.[3] Burgeoning profits, standardization of beauty practices, and relatively lax or poorly regulated legal frameworks for beauty supplies in many countries are some of the reasons why cosmetic emporiums have exponentially grown in the last decades, in terms of size as well as presence across borders and regions.[4] Other factors include the increased presence of women in the work market in emerging countries, the role of mediatization in private life, for instance, through photos of otherwise undocumented intimate moments, and the complex and multilayered relation between new marketing devices and branding strategies targeted for the presumed needs of each generation and cultural context.[5] In general terms, media outlets have played a vital role in the promotion of beauty and skincare products, targeting women to more degree than men.[6] Celebrities, movie stars of all statures, athletes, and other influential figures have lent or rather leased their faces to advertise what many consider to be the tools to attain an agreeable look, or at least, to be a step closer to the beauty canons of each time and space.[7] Cosmetics mirror idealizations about the human physiognomy and perceived instrumentality of strategies devised to deliver more attractive and healthier looks. Since preparations fluctuate across a continuum ranging from chemical and synthetic compounds to plant-derived, ethnobotanic, and artisanal formulas, cosmetics materialize imaginaries about nature and its properties for the care, maintenance, and improvement of physical appearance. At the same time, these are artifacts conditioned by the juxtaposition of understandings about femininity, masculinity, material culture, and knowledge. By proxy, cosmetics can be regarded as gendered epistemic artifacts created to embellish, target, and enhance the human body in one way or another.

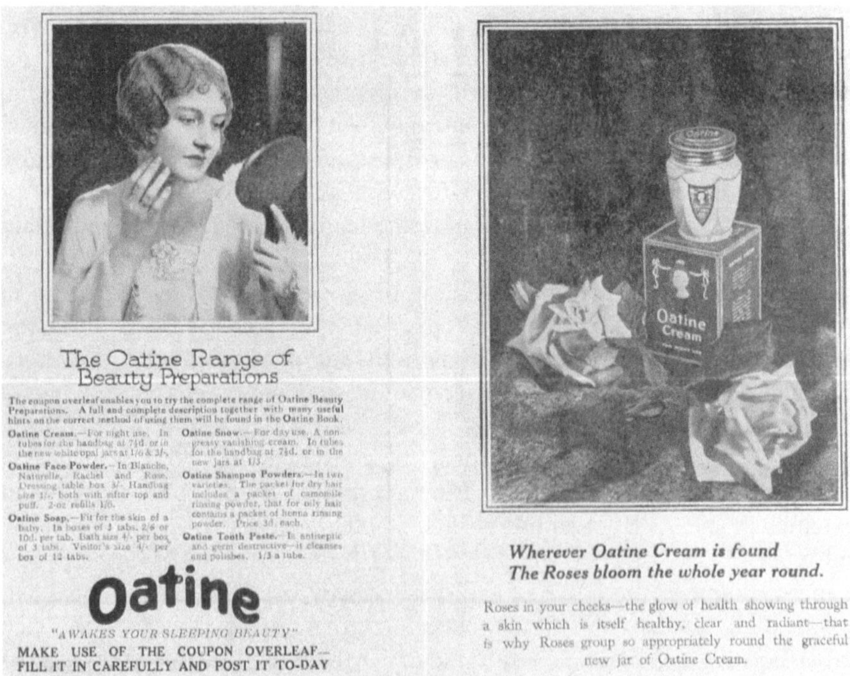

Figure 4.1 Picture of a Leaflet for Oatine Cream. *Source*: Wellcome Collection. Attribution 4.0 International (CC BY 4.0).

The main focus has laid upon the largest of the organs, the skin. Few parts of the human anatomy are as visual and culturally symbolic as the outer layer covering its entirety. Beyond its function of protecting the body, sensing the environment, regulating changes, and externalizing certain anomalies, the skin is often the receptor and working milieu of any attempt to improve one's aesthetic look. The voracious appetite for cosmetic preparations explains the widespread use of herbs, fruits, plants, barks, nuts, animals, and mineral extracts that civilizations have developed for thousands of years.[8] Routinary endeavors to decorate, maintain, restore, heal, and improve the most visible parts, such as the face, neck, and hands, have been the main concerns for both users and producers ever since the production of beauty care products became an industry. Advances in chemistry defined the technification of skincare in the nineteenth and early twentieth centuries,[9] but formulas and homemade mixtures based on common ingredients, such as oatmeal, honey, or rose water, have never ceased to exist (figure 4.1). Reemerged interest in eco-friendly approaches has sparked interest in additive-free, plant-based formulas. Today, a tapestry of imagery and information about skincare innovations travel across networks of consumption ruled by popular culture, social media trends, and branding strategies responsive to changes in customers' attitudes and needs.

As a reaction to the so-called Green Beauty trend, in recent years, many companies have incorporated protocols and lines of products that take into consideration ecological concerns of their customers, most of which are targeted at women.[10] In a landscape dominated by the idea that natural ingredients cannot harm either humans or the environment, fruits, plant extracts, animal excretions, and even venoms, for instance, the one secreted by bees and snakes, have made their way into minimalist stylish jars or appealing playful sachets sold all over the globe. Notwithstanding, it is worth noting that there is nothing new about the use of ethnobotany for cosmetic purposes. Most civilizations across time have evolved methods to harness sources from the natural world to decorate, heal, and protect human skin.

While Assyrians, Babylonians, and Sumerians knew the effect of plants such as belladonna (*Atropa belladonna* L.), cardamom (*Elettaria cardamomum* L. Maton), and myrrh (*Boswellia sacra* Fluck),[11] Native Americans were acquainted with the potentialities of various techniques to produce body pigments of all sorts, applied for their aesthetic, semiotic, and functional value.[12] Besides the contested notion of race, the cultural symbolism of skin in social life is, above all, prominent in the pervasive and perhaps universal desire to retain a youthful appearance. Written sources have historically documented attempts of physicians, pharmacists, and chemists to produce remedies to alleviate and dissipate wrinkles.[13] Health professionals were in many ways beauty professionals. Two of the most prominent medical compendiums written in East Asia, for instance, include passages on recipes that can be used for aesthetic purposes. *Shennong Classic of Herbal Medicine* (神農本草經 /神农本草), commonly known as *Shennong Bencao Jing* (compiled around 200–250 CE), mentions, among others, the anti-aging properties of Chinese wax gourd seed (冬瓜子) (*Semen benincasae hispidae*) and the efficacy of silkworm (僵蠶) (*Bombyx batryticatus*) to treat speckles.[14] In like manner, *Dongui Bogam* (동의보감 / 東醫寶鑑), a Korean materia medica classic written by Heo Jun during the Joseon Dynasty, and published in 1513, includes entries on 52 herbs with skincare properties.[15] Across Asia, some folk remedies recorded centuries ago are still used, such as rice water.

Biomedicine and advances in chemistry and pharmacology have not entirely replaced ancient wisdom, perhaps, because it is anchored in heritage, cosmologies, and traditions passed on from generation to generation. A sense of attachment seems to define the relation between societies and knowledge that has stood time. A case in point is the special attention South Korean cosmetic companies have recently devoted to the renaissance of traditional Korean holistic medicine, or Hanbang (한방), as one of many sources of inspiration for the ambitious development of innovative lines of skincare products that appeal to local and international markets.[16] A move that can, of course, also be regarded as a convenient, lucrative business decision at a time when customers make demands for green cosmetics.

Known for cutting-edge and innovative formulas, for instance, a facial mask containing charcoal, bubbles, and berries (figure 4.2), South Korean brands have managed to conquer customers across the globe. This has happened hand in hand with the seducing effects of *hallyu* (한류) or The Korean Wave. An observed increase in popularity of Korean cultural production has been credited to the spread of television series and music bands.[17] As a trend, *hallyu* has been primarily prompted by the circulation and consumption of visual culture and the unhindered outreach of contemporary mediascapes. Latin America has not been immune to this global phenomenon, and Korean cosmetics have been embraced positively since their incursion into the continent in the early 2000s. The presence of Korean cosmetic companies is global and is increasingly growing. Through flagship stores and e-commerce channels, major K-Beauty (Korean cosmetic industry) key players have opened stores or created networks of distribution in Brazil, Chile, Colombia, Mexico, and Paraguay. Ingredients formerly unknown to Latin Americans as possible components for skincare formulas have progressively expanded the palette of preparations adopted by consumers of cosmetics across the region. More importantly, their presence denotes and underlines the fact that commercial endeavors can result in epistemic exchanges.

Albeit partially, Korean ideas, traditions, and practices that involve nature as an agent to treat, heal, and improve the human skin have become part of the

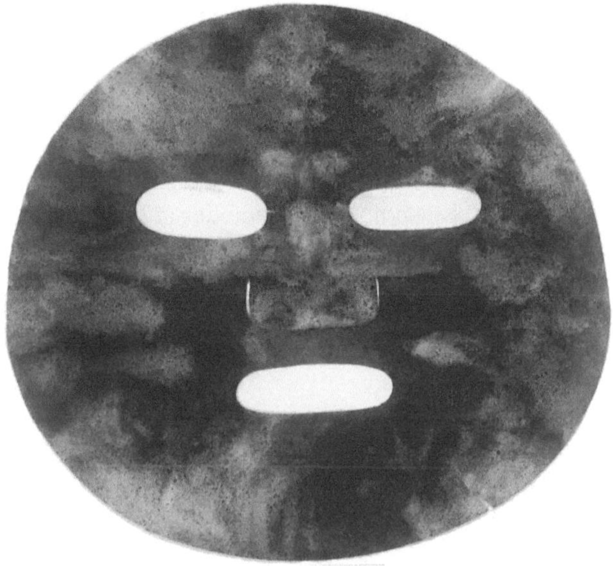

Figure 4.2 Korean Facial Mask Containing Carbon Residues, Sparkling Bubbles, and Berries. *Source*: Photo by author.

repertoire of many users in countries on the other side of the Pacific. A closer look reveals that some of the commonalities shared by South Korea and Latin America have facilitated these exchanges. Clear-cut gender stereotypes and roles, heavily grounded in patriarchal discourses, inform the set of ideas about the position of women and men. Furthermore, in both regions, there is interest in skin-whitening formulas, reflecting a preference for light complexions, and audiences embrace informal media formats as outlets to pass down information about herbal lore and traditional home remedies.

KNOWLEDGE, EXCHANGES, AND IMAGES

Images play an important role in mobilizing ideas about the intricate relation between beauty, health, and the natural world. Profiting from web syndication, formats such as video blogs and filmed tutorials have become common tools to dispense advice, tips, and recommendations about the medicinal properties of skincare products. Open source platforms, YouTube in particular, have enabled vloggers (video bloggers) to create their own content and disseminate it, mostly unhindered, across personalized channels.[18] The individual, informal, unregulated, and uncertified aspect of this production of media aligns with the relatively lenient regulations surrounding the promotion of cosmetics,[19] particularly problematic for three reasons. First, claims made by cosmetic companies for marketing purposes remain in many cases outside surveillance of (inter)national food and drug agencies in terms of verifiability and accuracy. Homemade media content risks echoing and amplifying the information provided by the brands, at times, despite the questionability of its veracity. Second, since cosmetics are often used with relative continuity and, in combination with other consumables, even more so than other substances, consumers, and societies at large might benefit from having exact information about their efficacy, suitability, side effects, long-term impact, and environmental footprint—another aspect often neglected in media content produced to review or promote cosmetics. Third, the notion of naturality serves not only as a background to contextualize the advertisement of green cosmetics but also as a catalyzer for the production of communicational spaces where information dissemination is deformalized, simplified, informalized, and democratized, in the sense that knowledge exchanges do not necessarily rely on diffusion of facts, revised data, scientifically gathered evidence, or literature-based observations. Since mass audiences have a burning interest in health- and beauty-related issues, nevertheless, exposure of viewers to visual culture production on the topic is quite widespread, either in the form of social media posts, video blogs, or a combination of both.

In the process, a large amount of visual content is produced on the perception and tropes surrounding the healing properties of nature for cosmetic purposes. Although much of the content operates as an advertisement in the form of firsthand users' reviews, advice from self-appointed experts, or promotional ads disguised in personal experience accounts, it is impossible to ignore that part of what is shared mirrors pieces and elements of local epistemologies, epistemic regimes, century-old folklore, informal systems of knowledge, and local common beliefs. Furthermore, beyond their scope, vlogs dedicated to address concerns about aesthetic and beauty-related issues tend to dispense advice about general well-being. Often, the content varies according to the gender of the target audience. Recommendations about how to obtain the ideal body weight, deploy stress-managing strategies, implement spirituality as a tool for inner beauty, and prevent undesirable medical conditions are some of the many topics discussed by health and beauty vloggers across the Internet.

Ariana Bonita (아리아나 보니따) is one of them. Described by viewers on YouTube and Instagram as a Latin Korean beauty influencer, she has gained notoriety for creating content in Spanish. From her native South Korea, Ariana's vlogs address a variety of subjects that range from healthy snacks to fitness routines, nutritional supplements to be taken during pregnancy, and descriptions of aspects of Korean daily life that might differ from those of the Spanish-speaking countries where many of her followers live. Above all, Korean cosmetics, innovative ingredients for the care and cure of the skin, home remedies, and recommendations on how to preserve a good appearance and good health are the central themes. Ariana's vlogs and posts combine product placement images with photos of various moments, rituals, and practices of her daily life. Her suggestions include massaging one's teeth with mashed strawberries to whiten them, eating tomatoes to dissipate cravings, or dissolving artichoke powder in water for better digestion. Besides digestive issues, female subscribers express in their comments the usefulness of routines to whiten their skin, a request accommodated by the diligent vlogger, who overtly explains the social role of light complexion in her home country. Fair skin and an attractive waistline are popular lines of inquiry in Ariana's social media outlets. Female followers, mostly, ask for specific information about Korean diets and Korean food items that can be ingested to lose weight. Studying the comments, there is a certain level of consensus among viewers that Koreans eat more naturally and therefore look young and slim. Hence, posting content on innovations in the landscape of healthy food supplements, such as moringa, and drinks containing calamansi (*Citrus x microcarpa*) to improve the skin and keep it in good balance is well-received by audiences.[20] Beyond the particulars of Ariana's beauty and health tips, through the comments from subscribers, it becomes clear that she introduces elements of Asian material culture and heritage unknown to many Latin Americans. Calamansi, a citrus hybrid also known as Philippine lime/lemon or calamondin, for instance, prompts a sense of strangeness and marvel. Similarly, the use of a flower stem as food, such as lotus root, *yeonguen* (연근), does not go unnoticed, reflecting in the process different conceptualizations of nutrition, food heritage, and health.

Ariana's posts tap into the sense of novelty and the pursuit of information and entertainment her channel's subscribers seek. Her vlogs, like many other hybrid media cultural artifacts, epitomize the role of digital spaces as a milieu of exchanges on a global scale. Despite their presumed superficiality and triviality, informal and artisanal homemade visual artifacts, such as video vlogs, encapsulate epistemic exchanges through formats and subjects that escape the rubrics of formalized knowledge dissemination outlets. Through entertaining brief episodes, or staged photographs, audiences learn that in Ariana's world, nature and beauty are interlinked but not quite in the same way as it is in their immediate surroundings. Ever-evolving digital ecologies take on their suitable role as avenues to register and diffuse novelties across borders. Commenting on the constant flux of trends, commodities, and practices becomes a form of visual entertainment. Images alert to the fact that the relation between health and beauty in the twenty-first century relies on the notion that innovation is unavoidable in a capitalist system, where innovations underline the "fetish character of the commodity in its monopolistic peculiarity."[21] Consequently, a dialogue between vlogger and subscriber about the image of an exotic citrus fruit, such as calamondin, that allegedly does wonders for the skin revolves around ideas about its properties but ultimately also about its availability and commercialization as a commodity. There are many possible answers to the question, where can I buy it?

In an era of multilevel interconnectivity, one small or large community's ethnobotanical tradition has the potential (or risk?) to easily become part of a common body of knowledge. Neo-colonialism, economic interests, bioprospecting, and changes in prevailing tendencies have contributed, for example, to globalized overconsumption of avocado, quinoa, gooseberries, and amaranth as de rigueur superfoods, with consequences for vulnerable communities. In that sense, ingredients for the preparation of cosmetic formulas or remedies are no different. Under the umbrella of green innovation, readoption of long-forgotten or overlooked epistemic heritage, or revolutionary discoveries, raw materials with exotic names and painstakingly produced in far-flung destinations retain their status as commodities in the twenty-first century.

Fighting *Natural* Aging

Urgency to develop competitive products has prompted, for instance, the increased appetite for facial creams, lotion, serums, masks, and other formats of skincare consumables containing snail mucin. In their presumed capacity to alleviate, besides expression lines, skin conditions, such as acne, hyperpigmentation, and scars, snail mucin-based products can be considered to be cosmeceuticals. A term used to refer to cosmetics containing, health-enhancing bioactive ingredients, coined by Albert Kligman in 1984 but not recognized as a legal category or product classification.[22] In the case of snail mucin-based cosmetics, despite their capacity to affect, even if minimally, the function or structure of the human body, they are mostly regarded, at least from a regulatory perspective, as products intended to beautify and enhance attractiveness. Wrapped in bright pastel-colored, simplistic, but gleaming, and glossy jars and tubes, the content and function of these products denote the complex interconnection between nature, culture, and epistemic systems. On the one hand, these formulas concentrate the operationalization of knowledge about substances produced by living organisms (e.g., snails); on the other, they betoken the management of natural resources and the role of raw materials at the service of human pursuit for health and beauty, as it seems a perennial quest for improvement.

All along, cultural representations articulate and register the ways in which gender-oriented aesthetic canons inform the production of artifacts and ignite the propagation of visual tropes. #Snailmucin posts on Instagram lead to short videos, photos, infographics, reviews, and to the expected plethora of visual advertisement material that creatively lauds the benefits of the revered mollusk excretion in the human fight against imperfections and (natural) aging process of the skin. Saturation of images is indicative of the economy of visuals that distinguishes contemporary public discourse.[23] Recognition and visibility for commercial purposes presupposes the use of tools that enhance visibility, convince, and seduce, even in the face of facts. A major controversy erupted from an exposé broadcast in 2011 by MBC's investigative report show 달팽이 점액 (*Up to zero complaints*) on the limited amount of actual snail mucin, as opposed to snail mucin filtrate in skincare products, has not necessarily lead to the abolition of snail excretion derivatives. Snail-related substances are still used in a large number of South Korean cosmetic products. The iconicity of the local celebrities, and influential figures that contribute to the promotion of snail filtrate consumables, is in line with the originality of eye-catching label names, such as Mizon Snail Recovery Gel Cream, COSRX Advanced Snail 92 All in One, Luminositie Snail Essence Renewal, Íunik Snail Serum, and SeoulCeuticals Korean Skin Care Snail Repair Cream.

Albeit South Korean brands currently stand out for the prolific development and domination of the market for snail mucin derivatives, the first commercial use of the substance was patented in Chile in 1993. According to Fernando Bascuñán Dockendorff (1940–2017)—the founder of Elicina Cosmetics Ltd., the pioneer cosmetic brand behind the earliest attempt to commercialize snail mucin for cosmetic purposes—the discovery of the effect of the filtrate was accidental. In interviews and promotional material, Bascuñán Dockendorff consistently explained how some of his employees, operating a harvesting facility for edible land snails, noticed the impressive efficacy of the mucin in treating work-related scratches and wounds in hands and forearms.[24] The eventual development of a line of anti-aging and scar-improving creams took place, according to Elicina's former director, only after a rigorous study confirmed the efficacy of the snail filtrate. The outcome meant for the family business to transition from a snail farm into a global leading producer of snail mucin-based cosmeceuticals, directing the attention of South Korean companies toward this apparent novelty.

Registration of the patent did not mean that knowledge about the active bioingredients in snail excretions was new, as historic sources confirm that the benefits of mollusks to treat dermatological conditions have been known for centuries. Written texts certify that since antiquity, Ancient Greek and Early Byzantine civilizations saw in snails sources of curative treatments for skin conditions.[25] Preparations varied according to author, region, and purpose, but besides dermatological afflictions, snails were presumed to alleviate ulcers and other digestive system disorders. While external applications of mollusks were recommended for wounds and burns in Asia Minor, snails were seen as effective treatments for symptoms related to sexually transmitted diseases in East Asia. Important figures in the history of medicine, such as Hipocrates and Dioscarides, recommended the use of snails to treat skin-related annoyances. While the former one advised applying crushed snails to ameliorate inflammation, the second one endorsed their properties against bumps and warts, in particular, when burnt and dry.[26] In *De re medica*, Aulus Cornelius Celsus also extols the benefits of macerated snails for dermatological concerns, concentrating specifically on sores. By the same token, Pliny the Elder assigns a number of passages in *Naturalis Historia* to the pharmacological effectivity of mollusks as a targeted treatment for ulcers. Archival sources indicate the use of snails in Europe for remedial purposes was not uncommon in the seventeenth and eighteenth centuries, serving as the base for remedies to treat a series of ailments.[27] Interest in the curative potentialities of snails in publications dating from the late eighteenth and early nineteenth centuries implies that there was a certain acknowledgment of their medicinal properties in Europe. In like manner, most Oriental medicine compendiums have consistently reported on the health benefits from ingesting snails or applying snail-based compounds to localized parts of the body. Led by American and European research centers, studies conducted in the twentieth and twenty-first centuries have provided new insights into the possible pharmacological applications of snail mucin. The history of snail and derivatives for curative purposes indicates they have mainly been used to mitigate health-related concerns.

This has dramatically changed, and today, snail slime has become an iconic ingredient in the development of products that eliminate and reduce creases, expression lines, hyperpigmentation marks, visible scars, and rhytids.[28] Snail mucin fulfills the criteria of a natural ingredient that is only minimally processed and yet effective, according to the many brands behind their commercialization. Since green beauty standards stipulate awareness about the use of natural resources, potential customers show interest in knowing more about the processes of breeding, farming, collection, extraction, and general well-being of the animals. A key detail to contextualize the supply of the filtrate is the fact that snails excrete it under special circumstances that do not harm them, theoretically, in any way. Undisruptive external stimuli should suffice. In fact, producing mucin is a mechanism that enables snails to adhere to surfaces, protect their own skin from bacteria and strong UV rays, and prevent excessive drought due to overexposure to the sun. Even if snails are one of the most diverse land animals in the world, modern-day snail mucin used for cosmetic preparations is mainly extracted from garden snails (*Cornu aspersum*), advertised in some South Korean products as Chilean Black Snails. Ecological concerns have redefined the level of specificity of the information provided by cosmetic manufacturers, in terms of composition and efficacy.

Materials used to advertise snail filtrate-containing consumables stress the fact that they possess antimicrobial and antioxidant properties, in line with the conventions observed by many producers of cosmetics that underline the importance of prevention of possible threats.[29] Although the definition of skin condition is not straightforward, certain processes are customarily mentioned as damaging for those interested in pursuing a youthful appearance. Properties attributed to the mollusk's excretion align with the expectations of the lucrative anti-aging industry, targeted mainly at adult women, although anti-wrinkle products occupy a special place in the daily routine of millions of people of all genders. Favoritism of faces with a smooth and spotless complexion in images diffused invasively across mediascapes boosts furthermore the cultural capital of ageless bodies. Tutorials, vlogs, blogs, and social media reviews posted by customers serve as repositories of exchanges between influential figures, consumers, health gurus, and brand research and marketing teams.[30] As part of a coherent marketing strategy, infographics, ads, and campaign advertisement videos secure the diffusion of the technical terms that explain why snail mucin has such a positive impact on the skin. Snail slime is branded as a potent agent to prevent water loss on the dermis and to increase the replacement of dead skin cells. Snail slime serum contains hyaluronic acid, polypeptides, and glycolic acid, which are all elements customers look for in a product that claims to accelerate the production of collagen, restore skin dullness, and prevent the formation of wrinkles—a true cosmeceutical.[31] An animal gland secretion emerges as an effective *natural* weapon in a war against markers of *natural* aging processes.

The visual dimension of appearing "natural" involves creating the illusion not only that the essence of each ingredient has been kept but also that each component retains the rawness of its provenance. Thus, K-Beauty, as the Korean cosmetic industry is internationally branded, relies on images as much as it relies on the development and research of revolutionary products that imply newness without compromising pristine greenness. An amalgamation of old, new, and, for some, exotic additions—such as volcanic lava, fish eggs, pig collagen, propolis, and a considerable number of carefully curated plant extracts, exported to all corners of the planet—is undoubtedly expanding the definition of what a cosmetic actually is and what is made of.[32] A close interconnection between K-pop (Korean popular music) celebrities and K-Beauty (Korean cosmetic brands) advertisement campaigns becomes evident as famous singers and film stars extol the qualities of the products they use.[33] Not surprisingly, their loyalty to local Korean skincare innovations and how vocal they are about it can partially explain the popularity and sales of companies such as Innisfree and The Saem. Icons and products are unavoidably coupled through the prevalence of media spaces as catalyzers of trends that mobilize not only material goods (e.g., lipsticks) and cultural artifacts (e.g., soap operas) but also epistemic artifacts (e.g., Hanbang skincare formulas). Albeit, even if only partially, knowledge is transmitted through the materialization of objects that are developed as extension of intragenerational epistemologies, century-old praxes, and documented (even if orally) observations. In this sense, media acts as a tool to facilitate knowledge transfers, nonetheless, on the way in which a society regards the role of nature in the care and cure of the human body.

Visualizing Imaginaries and Commodities

Images that depict the instrumentality of nature in the procurement of health operate at the same time as repositories of information about attitudes and imaginaries held by their producers. A sense of manifoldness and heterogeneousness seems to distinguish the conceptualization of how and which objects immaculately ought to remain in their natural state in order to retain and maximize their medicinal properties. Attempts to create pictorial representations involve revealing inclusion and exclusion of elements, according to a certain set of characteristics and traits. Skillfully deployed visual framing strategies reveal that the relation between nature and health juxtaposes national identity, and national (self)-branding, as much as it reinforces stereotypical ideas about gender and an imagined exotic Other. In terms of their positive effect on the body, while Icelanders proudly elevate the purity of Icelandic water (see chapter 5), Koreans embrace raw materials from distant locations (e.g., Chile) or from local, but perceptually special settings (e.g., Jeju Island). In a quest to deliver the highest level of purity that could secure outstandingly superior raw ingredients, according to the ads, one South Korean company has found in Madagascar the last reservoir of pristine *Centella asiatica* plants, colloquially known as Indian pennywort, gotu kola, or tiger grass across East Asia.[34]

On the surface, Centella Light Cleansing Oil or Skin1004 Madagascar Centella Hyalu-Cica Sleeping Pack appear to be average consumables, promoted as revolutionary cosmetic innovations through the use of references that enhance their appeal. The packages resemble similar products in the market, and the claims about effectivity are also in line with the expectations of the target buyers. The company behind their conceptualization Skin1004 is one of many international brands, headquartered along Seoul's Teheran-ro (테헤란로) (Teheran Boulevard), a hub of cosmopolitan globally oriented companies. The raw material, a plant known for centuries for its medicinal properties, is not a novelty either. Yet, there seems to be more to the marketing-driven strategic associations that ornate these jars, tubes, sachets, and bottles. According to the promotional video, the *Centella asiatica* plants collected in Madagascar make the products unique because they grow on the "oldest island on Earth," home to "200 million years of untouched nature." Even if the fickleness and transience of advertisement material trivializes its content or discourages its study in terms of attitudes and circulation of ideas, it does not fail to document, for instance, one possible set of notions about the natural world.

The collection of videos in English with Korean subtitles indicates the strategic decision of appealing to global markets while addressing the needs of local customers. A central message in the conceptualization of the campaign is that the wisdom behind the efficacy of the plants comes from the natives who have survived despite "facing cruel Mother nature generation after generation." Skin1004 underlines the importance of discovering the existence of *Centella asiatica* in such a pure and pristine state and, yet, quite far away from the unidentified international, presumably, Korean skincare products customers. The situatedness of the national and international in the context of health is reminiscent of how Koreans have historically responded to the marketing of medicines. As Suh (2018) has observed, "The changing relationship between the indigenous and the foreign, or the local and the universal, enables us to view the ways in which the identity of Korean medicine has been created and modified over time" (478). A conclusion that aligns with the view that branding strategies of Korean companies "reflect[s] simultaneously the complexities of prescriptive regimes of beauty from global and local consumer cultures."[35]

Nostalgic images of an idyllic, almost primigenial, and relatively forgotten corner of the globe reinforce the idea that the *cica* plants from Madagascar are one of a kind. The ads hide the fact that *Centella asiatica* is endemic to many more places and that it has been part of Malagasy traditional practices for a long time. In fact, *talapetraka*, as is known locally, played an important role in the treatment of leprosy, even if its accurate anti-leprosy agents were poorly understood.[36] In modern Madagascar, it is known not only for alleviating upset stomachs but also to complement or season meals. The international attention *cica* plants receive matters to many local communities where it represents sources of income for pickers, many of whom are women, working in the field from September to March. *Centella asiatica* is entwined in a network of exchanges at many levels, affected by decisions taken in Antananarivo and Seoul, and morphologically shifting roles and shapes as it circulates across the Indian Ocean. When *talapetraka* leaves the country, it ceases to be a product of the land, a herb or a revenue supply. It turns into a commodity and, eventually, an ingredient for cosmetics that, as the texts on the packaging state, quenches the thirst for the imagined or presumed properties of untouched Mother nature.

EMBODIMENT OF GENDERED IMAGINARIES

Beyond its semiotic and pictographic value, packaging of cosmetics and cosmeceuticals also holds value as a reflection of the social, rather than therapeutical, function of the products they contain. Preparations, formulas, and serums ultimately emerge from combinations of ingredients expected to improve physical appearance, as opposed to mitigate or heal serious health conditions that demand intervention. Commodities as objects that respond to the fetishism for novelty, encouraged and sustained by capitalist agendas, not only become raw materials for profit-generating end-products but also instruments to maintain gendered beauty regimes. The use of bioactive ingredients is indicative, ideally, of knowledge about their efficacy and effect on the human body, and the diversity of substances and methods implies that societies understand and relate to nature differently. It is logical since each community has interacted with the specificity of its immediate landscapes, topographies, and ecosystems, weaving distinct histories and cultural practices that through observation and experience have forged bodies of information particularly relevant to each one of them. Knowledge transfers about preparations for cosmetic purposes elucidate the universality of contrivances that embody aesthetic idealizations. Cultural representations, just as modern-day cosmetics, emerge from the appliance of technology, amplifying the set of ideas and imaginaries behind their production in the first place. Beauty products promoted mainly to target women denote the gendered dimension that transverses the creation of cultural artifacts and their role in consolidating notions of masculine, feminine, and binary identities.

Identity is an important notion to understand the centrality of nature as a concept with a social leverage in all cultures. No society can afford to endure without understanding its surroundings, and no society fails to recognize, at least partially, the role and interplay of biological genders in securing the survival of the species. Even if cosmetics might be considered trivial artifacts with limited potential as epistemic contraptions, or perhaps too superficial in scope, a valid observation is that an anti-wrinkle cream marketed for women entering menopause mirrors simultaneously ideas about gender, health, technology, and naturality. The particular case of green cosmetics in South Korea and Latin America, for instance, can be studied from a demographic perspective, focusing on the incursion of women in the workforce and their increased social presence and disposable income.[37] In broader terms, the commercialization of beauty is closely followed and conditioned by the evasive presence of images and media exposure, exerting influence on attitudes, health identities, and presumably *healthy* identities.[38] Anti-aging cosmetics, manufactured with natural ingredients, align comfortably and conveniently with a time in which human life span increases in a planet seriously affected by an environmental crisis of unprecedented scale. Female customers remain in the position of main potential targeted receptors of products designed for them to conform with beauty canons, while being attentive to their own health and what the manufacture of skincare consumables means for the planet.

Cosmetics are products of cultural, social, economic, political, and epistemic processes and at the same time, they are part of networks of artifacts that encompass the fringe between aesthetics, health, aspirations, and safety. Consumers trust what they perceive as extensions of nature to beautify their appearance while allegedly contributing to the well-being of the largest of their organs: the skin. The biological outer layer of the human anatomy is receptacle of substances, formulas, and combinations that purportedly respond to the needs of each user. Women use more cosmetics than men. Female consumers constitute the main target audience for images and packages that visually seduce and convince them. A plethora of interests lie behind the commercialization of beauty. The engine behind the mobilization of skincare products globally has a lot to do with large multinationals and lax regulations for cosmetics. Their size might affect their logos in the coming decades. Changes in attitudes, ecological awareness, and, to a certain degree, greenwashing ideologies have repositioned the popularity of artisanal health-enhancing products. New "small" brands are emerging (daughter companies of larger corporations) in response to this trend, although some other are not pretending to be small, they are.

The Machinery of Beauty

Murals on the walls displaying argan trees (*Argania spinosa*), locally known as ⴰⵔⴳⴰⵏ / أركان, decorate some of the cooperatives where local women come together to produce facial creams, shampoos, soaps, scrub masks, and enhanced oil compounds.[39] Morocco is proud of its endemic tree and its properties. Locals are equally proud of transforming their celebrated natural resources into an end-product recognized by avid customers all over the world. "Argan oil can be eaten or used on the skin," explains the shop owner and co-manager of one of the artisanal workshops while she offers samples of the different items they manufacture.[40] There are no signs of actual trees that colorfully ornament the streets of Essaouira, sale catalogs, or the jars of the argan oil cosmetics.[41] The essential raw materials are the nuts, but the iconicity of the tree retains its symbolic value across the various stages of production, distribution, and commercialization. In some products marketed in Europe, arabesque-themed fonts and diagrams serve as references to the provenance of the popular substance.

Argan oil is less accessible as an ingredient in food products outside Morocco (except in specialized shops) even if the production of most co-opts include comestibles, such as cooking oil, spreads, sweeteners, and candies. Local communities consume it in salads, couscous, and as a dip, and the oil has a unique place in Moroccan and Amazigh cuisines and diets. Mostly employing female workers, many small-scale argan oil processing firms are (or emerged as) indirect extensions of programs propelled by European cooperation agencies.[42] Through incentives, training, and community participation campaigns, argan oil co-ops have played a role in creating work opportunities for local women. The working model is new, but the use of argan oil is a century-old tradition in regions such as Merrakec-Asfi. The labor conditions of the employees working in the industry have been an object of discussion in media outlets and academic scholarship.[43] Although there seem to be unresolved issues, many celebrate that there are new sources of income for a quite fragile segment of the local population. The trees are indexical of an industry that improves not only economic prospects but also of a better ecosystem. *Argania spinosa* is fundamental to retain the stability in the area, contributing to the hydrologic systems that feed the aquifers, preventing the risks of soil erosion and protecting landscapes from the rampant spread of desertification across North Africa. As the helpful and eloquent co-op employee points out, "The trees are also very good places to hide from the sun during the hottest months of the year." While the women sit on the ground and process the compacted lumps that result from separating the oil from its residues, it is unavoidable to notice all signs are in French and English. I do not refer only to the labels on the jars being sold but to the general linguistic landscape of the women's cooperative facility. Arabic and Amazigh are absent from walls and cosmetic packaging. The trees are also absent. An argan oil extraction machine (figure 4.3) converts *Argania spinosa* kernels into dense, compact lumps that separate the fruit from the precious substance. Perhaps another type of machine sieves the local culture (local flavors and languages) from spaces destined to sound and look international.

A special place is dedicated to the guests visiting the cooperative and an equally characteristic room is assigned to the machine that makes all this possible. The hydraulic oil press is not very large. Nonetheless, every member of the small firm appears to appreciate the efficient and vital role the press plays in the production of the argan oil cosmetics and consumables that generate income. As it appears, in some cases, a distinction is made between the women harvesting the nuts and those maneuvering them and turning them into exportable goods. Equal demarcations are noticeable between the products sold to local Moroccans and those waiting to reach overseas markets. Products destined for the national market, according to some informants, make less distinction between specific conditions and are prone to prefer oil

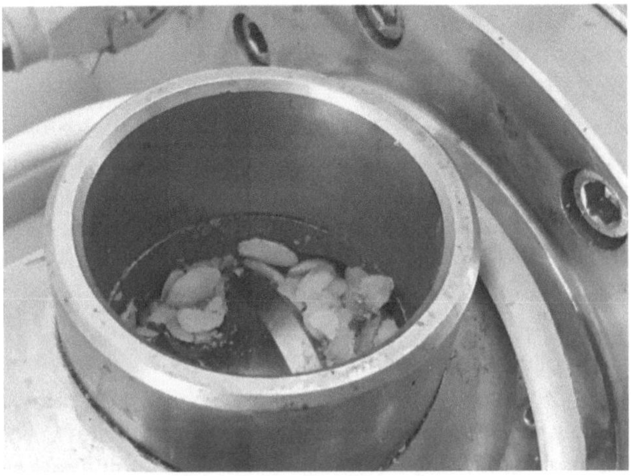

Figure 4.3 Argan Oil Extraction Machine. *Source*: Photo by author.

that does not contain any other ingredients. Even after confirming with locals, it is not always clear when argan oil consumables are primarily manufactured to be exported. They do confirm their preference for "clean argan oil with no extras." French is the lingua franca in Morocco and only on the basis of linguistic references, it would not be possible to discern between products and their envisioned markets. Back to the cooperative, the guide clarifies that foreigners are those predominantly visiting the shop. A few stay longer (something the cooperative workers visibly regret), follow the process, ask questions about the manufacturing and marketing techniques, and show interest in the technical aspects of creating artisanal cosmetics. The cooperative is a milieu of entrepreneurship, agency, and, possibly, means to create common good, for the employees, harvesters, and those purchasing items that purportedly can benefit their skin.[44] Questions about the degree of empowerment the argan oil create remain unanswered.[45] It is not only a matter of improving one's dermis. A number of creams are actual antieczema and anti-psoriasis preparations. There are many types of dermatitis and various degrees of severity of psoriasis, further subdivided into many types, all having in common, the frustration that accompanies having a condition for which there is no cure.[46] In this sense, cosmeceuticals permeate into territories that can become problematic for those who do not use facial or corporal compounds exclusively in the pursuit of gaining a rejuvenated, invigorated, or more attractive appearance. The co-op salesperson comments on how popular the "antieczema creams" are, along with the formulas against "dark circles" which occupy a special corner of the shelves. As the descriptions read, jars of argan oil essences combined with, for instance, lemon, arnica, jasmine, orange, and aloe vera are ideal to treat different kinds of skin problems. From greasy to dry skin, the compendium of combinations and formulas targets any possible customer in the pursuit of restoring, nourishing, improving, rejuvenating, and caring for her or his skin.

A shift in visuality has taken place with the advent of cosmetics in an era in which images permeate every aspect of private and public life. Materialization of attitudes through objects and cultural representations available to us indicates paradigm changes have taken place in many respects. Ideas about what health means and how to preserve it have evolved. The circulation and modification of canons to express ever-changing views bear testament to the impermanency of consensus about practices envisioned to cure and care for the body. A position that seems not to have mutated much is the human tendency to assume there is a connection between the presence of visibly exposed skin-deep markers and an internal, good health state. The biological borders of the body allegedly manifest, echo, show, and reveal a person's good or bad physical condition. Judging from comments on social media and the echo chamber carefully engineered by the apparatus of consortia behind the industries of advertisement, communication networks, and beauty products manufacturers many assume, claim, or promote that good appearance and healthy appearance come hand in hand. Studies show there is a psychological connection between, on the one hand, a person's (self)perceived beauty, skin texture, and color and, on the other, perception and assumptions about her own or someone else's medical condition. An added element to this equation is the set of connotations linked to the axiom schemata surrounding *nature* as a concept, physical place, system, nucleus, inspiration, reservoir, illusion, or utopia.

NOTES

1. Stewart (2017).
2. The nexus emerges in the form of a cross-cultural phenomenon (Eggerstedt et al., 2020; Hamid El Khoreiby, 2021; Wu et al., 2022) that fuels unrealistic expectations among potential consumers (Jung, 2018; Eagle and Hay, 2020), turning them into *patients* of paradoxical, complex, and unnecessary procedures (Lee, 2018; Wang et al., 2020; Bonell et al., 2021).
3. Danziger (2019).
4. Jeacle (2006).
5. One strategy that encompasses the notions of beauty and nature is the emphasis placed on appearing natural. However, a natural look risks becoming in itself a product (Smith et al., 2021).
6. Findings reveal similarities across the globe, in countries such as Bulgaria (Ghodsee, 2007), China (Barnes, 2004), Czech Republic (Rábová, 2015), Egypt (Mangal et al., 2021), France (Antioco et al., 2012), India (Ravikumar, 2012; Sultana,

2021), Iran (Shafeai and Sijanivandi, 2019), Japan (Barnes and Yamamoto, 2008), Kenya (Alubala, 2018), Morocco (Hamelin et al., 2018), Pakistan (Fatima and Lohdi, 2015), Peru (Urrutia Gómez, 2015), and Spain (Díaz Soloaga and Muñiz Muriel, 2011).

7. Bai (2018).

8. Stewart (2017).

9. Blanco-Dávila (2000).

10. Studies have identified ecological awareness, avoidance of chemicals, health concerns, generational traits, and aversion toward pollution as the main factors behind the Green Beauty trend (Matić and Puh, 2016; González-Minero et al., 2018; Thukaram, 2016; Al-Haddad et al., 2020; Kartawinata et al., 2020; Pop et al., 2020; Dini and Laneri, 2021; Sharma et al., 2021; Singhal and Malik, 2021; Tewari et al, 2021).

11. López (2007).

12. Dupey García and Vázquez de Ágredos Pascual (2019).

13. Benbow-Buitenhuis (2014).

14. Wang (2003); Hu (2017); Yuan (2020).

15. Gayoung et al. (2020).

16. The rise of *Hanbang* is having an impact on the perception of health as the set of biosocial practices that can nevertheless be attentive to the historically charged contexts in which it operates (Han, 1997; Han et al., 2005; Ma, 2010; Kang et al., 2019).

17. Korean pop music (K-pop) and soap operas have been instrumental in this process (Choi and Maliangkay, 2015).

18. Studies show vloggers (can) exert influence on viewers in terms of health- and beauty-related issues (Berryman and Kavka, 2017; Parnell, 2017; Nurvia and Sarasati, 2020; Mäkel et al., 2021; Xu et al., 2021).

19. De Regt, Montecchi, and Lord Ferguson (2019).

20. On studies about its properties, see, Yahya et al. (2014); Lv et al., (2015) ; Chen (2017).

21. Haug, 1986, 42.

22. Rohini (2002), Mukta and Adam (2010), and Brandt et al. (2011) discuss how denotations and connotations of the term fluctuate according to the context.

23. Szendy (2019).

24. According to the official website: "Elicina did not come into existence the way many other skin care products do. This cream originated on a snail farm in Chile, when the workers who handled the snails realized that minor cuts and abrasions on their hands healed much more quickly than was average, and that their skin always felt soft and smooth. It was found that the Helix Aspersa Muller snail secretions were the secret behind the healthy skin that had the ability to heal quickly. Further research on this special ingredient resulted in the birth of the Elicina Cream, which is a topical treatment used to treat a number of skin conditions and also as an anti-aging substance. After registering and patenting the process in which Elicina is made before The World Organization of Intellectual Property in Geneva Switzerland, in 1995 they launched the product to the South American market. Since its early beginning and with little publicity Elicina turned into a total success based exclusively on

the benefits experienced by the people that tried the cream. Shortly after Elicina was launched to global markets, and shortly became, thanks to the beneficiaries in the fight against strecth [*sic*] marks, skin burns, wrinkles age and sun spots, in a product of worldwide acceptance and success" (Elicina Official Site, 2020)

25. Figuier (1840), Philip (1864), Marchant (1902), Reutter (1915), and Voultsiadou (2010) confirm the use of molluscs as part of skincare routines since antiquity.

26. Voultsiadou, 2010.

27. Bonnemain (2005).

28. The emergent attention and applicability of snail mucin can presumably be traced to the patent (WO1992015276A3) filed by Rafael Abad Iglesias, entitled *Therapeutic and Cosmetic Compositions for Treatment of Skin* (1991).

29. On the properties of snail mucin, see, Tsoutsos et al. (2009), Kim (2015), No (2015), Pitt et al. (2015), Zhoh (2016), Cilia and Fratini (2018), Gentili (2020), and Nguyen (2020).

30. Wang and Lee (2021) have demonstrated the impact of influencers in promoting K-Beauty products among Chinese consumers.

31. Snail-based serums, even if they go through in vitro and in vivo mandatory testing stages, remain outside the regulation protocols that the Korean Food Administration stipulates for pharmaceuticals (Juhász et al., 2018). Although dermatologists were among the first in importing formulas with snail filtrate as main natural precursor, cosmetic products containing the substance have not been approved within the category of topical medications (Kim, 2008).

32. Shin (2019).

33. Wang and Lee (2021).

34. Nguyen, Masub, and Jagdeo (2020).

35. Seo et al., 2020, 613.

36. See Rasoanaivo et al. (2018) for more on the history of *talapetraka* in Madagascar and Reunion.

37. As well as in many other countries around the world. Green cosmetics production respond to sustainability concerns, environmental awareness (e.g., animal welfare), and the notion that personal values play a part in the production of the skincare consumables. Generational differences matter in terms of reception of these products (Liobikienė and Bernatonienė, 2017; Huy, 2021; Morganti et al., 2021; Patnaik et al., 2021; Sharma et al., 2021; Silva et al., 2021).

38. Singh and Singh (2011) observe that humans might have possibly evolved attractiveness assessing mechanisms, which suggest that arbitrariness or culturally constructed canons do not always account for the health-beauty linkage applied to women. A valid observation is that these canons can also be seen as "beauty regimes."

39. There is a tradition of using argan oil for cosmetic products, mostly limited to treat dry skin, acne, rhytids, dermatitis, and psoriasis (Charrouf and Guillaume, 1999, 2011).

40. Several studies have confirmed the therapeutical properties of argan oil, specifically through its consumption as part of human diet (Drissi, 2004; Cherki et al., 2006; El Monfalouti, 2010; El Abbassi, 2014; El Midaoui et al., 2016; Goik et al., 2019: Kharbach et al., 2021).

41. Although the co-operative granted me permission to mention their name openly in the book, I restrain from doing so.

42. The argan-oil-producing model has faced criticism mainly by those who argument that in the twenty-first century "labor struggles require more collaborative types of organization if they are to resist the global pressures that deepen poverty and informalization" (Meagher, 2019: 92).

43. See, le Polain and Lambin, 2013; Biermayr-Jenzano et al., 2014; Meagher, 2019; Rosengren, 2020.

44. Guillaume and Zoubida (2011) note that the oil has medicinal properties in the sense that it shows antiproliferative and antidiabetic activity, cancer preventive agents, and beneficial impact on the cardiovascular system. Yet, besides short-term anti-sebum activity, "cosmetic properties attributed to topical (beauty) oil are primarily based on traditional claims and have little scientific backing" (276).

45. Some scholars do not see the argan oil industry as a route toward empowerment of women or implementation of fair labor rights that disrupt hierarchical commodities chain where bottom-up programs fail to solve the root of inequality (Biermayr-Jenzano et. al, 2014 ; Meagher, 2019).

46. Dermatitis has effects on the daily life of millions of people, affecting them in profound ways, as shown by Blome (2016), Hill et al. (2016), Holm et al. (2016), Koszorú et al. (2019), and Kwak and Kim (2017). On the effect of severe psoriasis on quality of life, see Finley et al. (1995), Reich et al. (2014), Çakmur, Hülya and Derviş (2015), Yang (2015), Petraškienė (2016), Sarkar et al. (2016), and García et al. (2017).

Part III

SITES OF NATURE

Chapter 5

Topological Panaceas

This chapter delves into the topological (related to geo-cultural spaces) underpinnings that inform the notion of health in visual culture. Since many societies understand corporal well-being beyond the connotation of the presence/absence of disease or injury, they are creating conditions by which spaces participate in the promotion of healthiness. The belief that human-inhabited landscapes can operate as therapeutical, medicinal, remedial, and curative sites is not new. While for certain communities, the implementation of innovative projects is the basis of healthier lifestyles, for others, their territories are in essence intrinsic components of their well-being. Visual cultural artifacts suggest, for some nations, health has a topological dimension. Images contained in, for instance, documentaries, fictionalized narratives, brochures, street signs, food packaging, and websites express how their creators understand the topologies of health. These pictorial representations also provide cues about the attention devoted to aspects such as sanitation, hygiene, cleanliness of open spaces, public health, and general well-being.

Environmental concerns, intensified by the current sanitary and ecological crises, have prompted the increased emergence of media productions that address the relation between living organisms and their habitats. It is not only a matter of interest. For many communities across the world, the deterioration of ecosystems is having a direct impact on their daily lives. This concern is expressed visually. From YouTube vlogs to Tiktok short videos, graffiti in open spaces (e.g., "eco-graffiti"),[1] sarcastic images on t-shirts and ideograms on trash bins, and the dangers of an ailing planet are becoming prominent visual themes. Media outputs of various formats are registering the deployment of innovative social and economic projects to construct healthier landscapes, promote eco-friendlier lifestyles, and minimize humans' footprint on the planet.[2] Pictorial representations are documenting and contributing to make audiences more aware about the importance of preserving natural ecosystems, among other reasons, because it is the healthy thing to do.[3] Visuals are also appearing as responses of small communities to the fear of becoming collateral damage of an ecological disaster caused by more powerful countries.[4] Everything happens somewhere. The notion of space certainly applies to the dynamic between species and their surroundings. Human migrations explain our current presence in all corner of the globe and give an idea of the diversity of landscapes in which nations have built their homes. Ecosystems are as varied as ontological spectrums. The various topologies and their components have determined the sense of bioclusivity of the inhabitants in their continuous pursuit to live and thrive in those territories. As a crucially vital substance for all living organisms, water occupies a place in each culture. In this chapter, specifically the first section offers a discussion on the aquatic healthscapes in Iceland and the second focuses on the centrality of topologies in Okanagan medicine.

AQUATIC HEALTHSCAPES

The climatic, geological, and hydrological conditions of Iceland have reshaped the relation of its inhabitants with their environment ever since the island became a human settlement in ca. 870–874. An iconic swimming pool, Snorralaug (Snorri's Pool), has a special place in the Icelandic imaginary and list of heritage sites. It is perhaps not big in size (4 meters in diameter), but it has a grand history, nonetheless because it served as a bathing ground to the celebrated poet and politician Snorri Sturluson, the presumed author of *Egil's Saga* and possibly compiler/author of *Prose Edda*. Located in Reykholt (West Iceland), Snorralaug is plausibly the oldest human-made hot spring in the country. The relatively small bathing site links past and present in interesting ways. On the one hand, Icelanders regard their medieval manuscripts, and books, in general, as highly esteemed treasures and monuments to their long and respectable literary tradition. Not many sites mentioned in the reputable *Landnámabók* (*Book of Settlements*), written around half of the thirteenth century, have survived. Only on this account, this is certainly a special place. On the other hand, Snorri's pool is also a symbolic reminder of another quintessential aspect of Icelandic culture: making use of public bathing facilities outdoors. Despite what many people think when they visit the country, the actual tradition of swimming regularly and spending time in hot tubs is not necessarily related to a custom brought in by the first settlers. The construction of outdoor pools dates from the twentieth century. Both Snorralaug and contemporary bathing facilities share in common the use of geothermal energy. Despite the small size of the nation (ca. 376,248 inhabitants) (2022), the network of bathing facilities is extensive and reaches all the corners of the island nation. Being surrounded by the cold North Atlantic, the presence of water in the collective imaginary manifests also in the weight of fisheries for the close-knitted society. The often-cited saying *lífið er saltfiskur* (life is salted cod), immortalized in Nobel Laureate Halldór Laxness's epic novel *Salka Valka*, gives an idea of the place of the sea in Icelandic history, culture, and survival. Directly and indirectly, water has undeniably provided sustenance to the local communities since settlement times.

Although *sund* is the literal translation of "swimming," its English correspondent misses the contextualization of the series of activities linked to the places where Icelanders swim. An important aspect of outdoor bathing sites in Icelandic culture is that everyone seems to agree on how healthy it is. Posters, televised campaigns, social media posts, brochures, and advertisements in public areas (e.g., bus stops) play a part in the visualization of *sund* as a health-enhancing practice.

In the aftermath of the restrictions imposed by the Icelandic authorities to manage the Coronavirus pandemic, local municipalities closed the swimming pools. Through social media and news outlets, Icelanders expressed how impactful the closure of the bathing facilities was on their daily lives. In an unprecedented way, the measurement meant a disruption in an important daily routine for many *sundgestir* (swimming pool visitors). An interviewee described the shutdown as a source of "kvöl og pína" (torment and pain).[5] As the saddened usual guests explain, Icelandic swimming culture revolves around physical activity, but also the pools, bathtubs, steam baths, and saunas as social venues. There were examples of regular swimming fellows meeting in other places over coffee to discuss and speculate, among other things, when the facilities would reopen again.

Icelanders do not necessarily go to their public swimming pools only to improve their condition. These outdoor bathing sites have an interactional element that occupies a special place in the social fabric of urban and rural areas across the country. Bathers enjoy sitting in hot tubs (*heitir pottar*) discussing trivial and serious subjects. As Jónsson and Rastrick (2017) observe, there is nevertheless a code to observe, in the Icelandic case, it "involves minimal touching. You do not greet each other with a handshake; a nod is sufficient; hot-tub conversations are general and impersonal, even between regular visitors" (13). While these exchanges take place, in the background and all around them, water is present everywhere in different states and temperatures. It appears in the form of vapor in saunas and steam baths, or simply as water carefully regulated to meet specific standards of hygiene. The time of year has an impact on the use of the swimming pools as sunbathing sites, recreational waterparks, or places of relaxation. The dark winter months enhance the contrast between cold and heat. Icelanders appreciate being able to spend long periods of time outside sheltered inside a heated swimming pool and an even warmer *pottur* (tub). There are hot tubs that can reach up to 44 degrees centigrade (approximately 112 degrees Fahrenheit). Some are deliberately built as meeting grounds for families, children of all ages, tourists, and the most avid group of visitors. These are senior guests who have recently or long ago reached the age of retirement. They are specially visible in the morning hours not just as regular guests but also as members of social groups that emerge around the swimming pools as socialization venues. Iceland is a small country and many of them might already know each other before they started meeting up regularly in the hot tubs or in the pool lanes. For senior citizens, going to *sund* is a matter of attending encounters with age-peers and embracing the possibility of exchanging thoughts, experiences, and knowledge; showing comradery and kindness; practicing their social skills and ability to entertain others and being entertained; and activating communicational competencies, bonding, and reaching levels of communion that they might not find anywhere else. It is hard to argue that the companionship experienced by many of the retirees coming regularly to the swimming pools does not have a positive impact on their physical condition and states of mind. Rising life expectancy in industrialized nations prompts questions about the need to create mechanisms to serve senior citizens and Iceland might have already had a formula that seems to work.

A valid observation is that if *sund* is not a many-century-old tradition, then it seems peculiar how engrained and implanted this practice is in Iceland.[6] Swimming pools emerged in parallel with the establishment of other institutions. In only a few decades, "Schooling and other forms of socialization have led to the population's familiarity with the pool environment facilitating enjoyment and mental and spiritual enhancement on multiple levels with people seeking comfort and physical enhancement" (Jónsson and Rastrick, 2017, 13). The starting point of the present-day swimming pools was also linked to the development and access to technology that could make it feasible to harness geothermal energy.[7] The techniques to pipe water allowed for the reimplementation of an epistemic practice Icelanders already knew. They were aware that the geological conditions of the volcanic topology could offer the possibility of creating networks of distribution of geothermally heated water.[8]

Historical records indicate that the actual swimming pools were preceded by a desire of many to learn how to swim.[9] A particularly useful skill in a country of sailors and fishermen.[10] The first-ever recorded course took place in 1821, under the direction of Jón Þórláksson Kjærnested in Reistarár (North Iceland), followed by regular courses taught in Reykjavik three years later.[11] Toward the end of the nineteenth century, in some cases earlier, several municipalities introduced incipient forms of swimming education.[12] Jónas

Hallgrímsson (1807–1845), poet, writer, naturalist, and important name in Icelandic literature was among the most prominent public figures to raise awareness about the importance of learning how to swim.[13] Perhaps the drowning of his own father motivated him to translate the first manual on the subject, *Sund-reglur Prófessors Nachtegalls* (*Professor Nachtegall's Swimming rules*) (1836), which played a role in popularizing the sport among his fellow countrymen.[14] In the preface of the manual, Hallgrímsson notes that by the second decade of the nineteenth century, according to his estimates, only six people in the whole country "sem væru sjálfbjarga, ef þeír lentu í polli, sem þeír náðu ekki niðr' í" (would be able to save themselves if they fell into a pond of which they were unable to touch the bottom) (1836, vi). Less than a century later, the parliament dictated that swimming was to become a compulsory part of the national school curriculum. Emphasis was placed on teaching younger generations how to swim.[15]

Dying underwater was not the biggest cause of concern though. In early twentieth century, the effect of the First World War and the impact of the Spanish Flu brought along implications that affected to a higher degree the geographically isolated, small, and impoverished nations. Iceland was one of them. From 1911 and for over four decades, Iceland struggled with the devastating effects of tuberculosis, experiencing at some point the decimation of its capital's population, Reykjavik, caused by the infectious disease.[16] The impact of tuberculosis, locally known as *berklar* (and earlier on, also as *tæring*), became a significant burden on the national health system.[17] The trauma left many scars in the social fabric of urban and rural areas, nonetheless, because there was no treatment. Through images and texts, printed media recorded the evolution of the disease at a social level, from its first signs to the arrival of pharmaceuticals developed in American and Italian labs. There are almost 5,000 entries mentioning tuberculosis in the Icelandic newspapers published between 1890 and 1955, the year effective medication had reached large numbers of the affected population. In a two-volume edition of a special magazine entitled *Berklavarnarblaðið* (*Tuberculosis Newspaper*), published in 1939 and 1940, Icelandic patients found a space to express their own experiences living with the disease. So did doctors and those working with the patients in Kristneshæli, the main TB sanitorium in the country. In one of the volumes, Jóhann J.E. Kuld writes:

> In connection with the nation's increased physical activity, there is a vital need to put in place, both in the countryside and in towns, bathhouses, where saunas would be practiced by the general public, as was customary here during the settlement age. Most health professionals and modern sportspeople have come to the conclusion after thorough research that the simple old Finnish-Russian bathhouse, which has been used in these two countries for a thousand years, is the lifeblood that modern culture must adopt. Our cousins, the Swedes, who are

> considered to be at the forefront as a cultural nation, are now in the process of changing their largest bathing places so that they are in line with the thousand-year experience of the Finnish-Russian bathhouse. (Kuld, 1939, 2)[18]

In the same vein, during an interview, renowned writer Þorbergur Þórðarson (1888–1974) paints an image of how tuberculosis had an impact on the local mindset. To the question why he started practicing sports outdoors, Þórðarson replied:

> I guess it had been somehow influenced by dr. Helgi Pjeturss. He ran mostly around town to stay in good health and was quite fierce, sometimes he would run with a lifting device in the air in each hand. But these walks, runs and outdoor activities were mainly caused by fear of tuberculosis, which back then spread like wildfire. And many considered a good advice against tuberculosis to be as active as possible, swimming and running. Dr. Helgi Pjeturss did so for decades, going and running into the sea or the pools every Lord's day and getting in shape, he certainly kept a physical good shape well into old age. (Bergmann, 1964, 8)[19]

Since bathing culture was steadily becoming part of the national ethos, there does not seem to be a direct link between the biosocial impact of tuberculosis and outdoor swimming. Yet, from a thematic prominence perspective, aquatic activities do become more visible as tropes in the discussion of health-enhancing routines in print media. The use of hot springs and bathing outdoors is mentioned in medicine-related sections of nineteenth- and early twentieth-century newspapers to urge readers to realize the benefits of outdoor bathing sessions, steam rooms, and sauna culture.[20] The authors, some of whom were doctors, praised aquatic activities for their contributions to human health. Finnish sauna tradition served as an example of a therapeutic and effective way of staying in excellent athletic condition and of strengthening the capacity of the lungs. The advice was to embrace outdoor bathing as a way to gain better health.

In modern-day Iceland, *sund* culture is visually present in promotional material in newspapers and magazines, primarily sponsored by state-run institutions and municipalities, posters hung in schools' buildings, references in popular culture outlets, and by-products of activities organized to promote outdoor bathing practices (e.g., concerts taking place in the swimming pools). One of the recent physical and digital posters used to create awareness about the benefits of swimming is the one used to promote *Syndum* (Let's swim), a campaign launched in 2021 (figure 5.1) to encourage Icelanders to swim even more.

The idea is to ask them to register the distance after each session and have the possibility of winning a prize. All the distances swum are summed

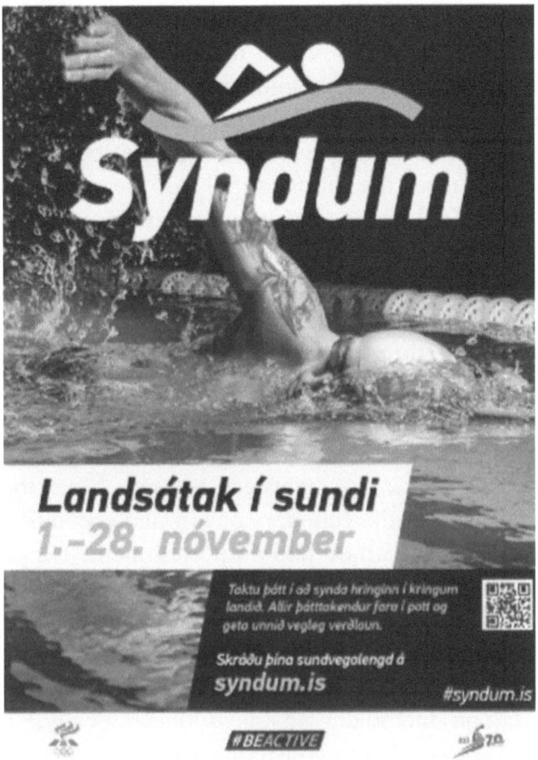
Syndum
Landsátak í sundi
1.–28. nóvember
Taktu þátt í að synda hringinn í kringum landið. Allir þátttakendur fara í pott og geta unnið vegleg verðlaun.
Skráðu þína sundvegalengd á
syndum.is
#syndum.is
#BEACTIVE

Figure 5.1 Poster of Syndum (Let's Swim) Promotional Campaign. *Source*: Courtesy and copyright of Íþrótta- og ólympíusamband Íslands/The National Olympic and Sports Association of Iceland.

up and displayed in terms of the number of kilometers that it takes to drive around Iceland. Users of the official website can also combine their registered distances with the number of meters they have run or biked. By the time the project ended, 1,652 participants had registered 13,344 sessions accounting for 15,360 kilometers, which are the equivalent of almost 12 trips around Iceland. Behind the creation of a prolific swimming culture lies the seemingly infinite access Icelanders have to geothermal energy. Bypassing the challenges faced by other countries in terms of energy resources, the geological conditions of the small volcanic island guarantee *sund* can presumably remain part of their *national DNA* for decades and centuries to come. The country has not only abundance of hot water. Along with Buthan and Guyana, Iceland also has one of the largest amounts of renewable internal freshwater resources per capita.[21] Icelanders are proud of their cold water and it is quite common to hear them say that *íslenskt vatn* (Icelandic water) is probably one (if not the) purest waters in the world.[22] Beyond the amour propre that the quality of the water evokes, it draws attention overseas and consequently, it has become a commodity sold abroad. Icelandic water in its "purest" state fills bottles easily available in cities like Paris or New York. In general terms, commercialization, branding, and a certain degree of fetishization inform many of the techniques used by multinationals that bottle and commercialize mineral water to meet the global supply of clean drinking water. At a national and international level, a reputation for immaculateness of the local water has found its way into visual representations that reflect how Icelanders and foreigners feel about the hydrological richness and general natural pristineness of the country. Besides its use for human consumption locally and abroad, some cosmetic manufacturers proudly state their preference for glacial Icelandic water in order to increase the skin hydrazination efficacy of their products. The colors used in promotional material resemble the milky blue shades and hues to promote the famous Blue Lagoon (*Bláa Lónið*), a manmade geothermal spa in southwestern Iceland. More than an emblematic site, it is a retreat and the founders of a brand specialized in cosmetics intended to encapsulate the allure and purported medicinal properties of the salts and algae of the place.

A connection between the water and what it means for Icelanders is probably best epitomized in a number of incidents surrounding foreign vegetables (2006, 2011, 2018). As in many other countries, in Iceland, the national flag is placed on a farming product to denote it is produced locally.[23] Concerns about eating healthier food have driven consumers to pay more attention to the use of national symbols as guidelines for the provenience and possibly quality of the items they purchase. Many want to eat nationally farmed consumables. On this account, it did not go unnoticed when local importers pasted the flag on the labels of foreign products, adding they were "þvegið úr íslensku vatni" (rinsed in Icelandic water).[24] One interpretation is that the distributors sought to imply that washing imported vegetables in the local water could be enough to *Icelandicize* them. Another reading is that by rinsing the food items locally, the distributors suggested their imported vegetables could reach the desired degree of cleanliness. In either case, the labeling strategy drew negative attention. Unionized farmers regretted the misuse of a visual strategy (Icelandic flag and accompanying text) as a tool to attract consumers by concealing the origin of the imported goods. The discussion surrounding the incident generated vociferous reactions. The special place Icelandic water occupies in the national soul was at the center of the debate. For many, it was a matter of honesty, misleading advertisement, lack of transparency, and above all, trust. The notion of cleanliness came to the surface and, specially, in terms of pesticides and agrochemicals. Due to the geographical position of the country, the absence of pests translates into the omission of herbicides and insecticides in almost all stages of farming.[25] Low levels of air pollution also recirculate in the form of cleaner agricultural goods. The controversy about the healthiness of local food and locally washed foreign vegetables ignited some Icelanders to discuss the role of water in agriculture. The debate prompted conversations about the biocultural function of hydrological resources in Iceland's national soul. In what looks as a reaction, Sölufélag garðyrkjumanna (Horticulturists' Sales Company), launched a campaign in 2018. It revolved around a series of images of consumers affectionately holding cucumbers, lettuce, and tomatoes and captioned with the question "Hvaða vatn fer í gegnum grænmetið þitt?" (Which water goes through your vegetables?).[26] Even if the campaign did not generate much polemic, the satirical undertone is added to a debate, once again, about the immaculateness of the local water.

The bottom line is that Icelanders are fully aware of the privilege of having almost endless access to the most vital natural resource for human life and which, besides, meets the highest international quality standards or what they perceive as *pure*.[27] I argue that this awareness reveals a deep connection with their aquatic resources and that it mirrors how they perceive water within their general sense of well-being and health. Water in Iceland is an important element of the country's healthscapes. Consumed internally, through drinking, farming, and fishing, and externally, through outdoor bathing, this indispensable substance denotes an embodiment of healthiness.

In terms of bioclusivity, I posit that water within the Icelandic mindset is part of their understanding of how nature plays a part in living well. The island nation has a relationship with its hydric resources that defines how they regard water as a constituent of their daily lives and as part of their culture. The story of how Iceland re-embraced the use of hot springs and swimming sites, after a many-century-long hiatus, exemplifies that the bioclusivity codes of a society are malleable, flexible, and adaptable. Visual culture has registered the changes and additions in terms of water as a resource, concept, substance, raw material, and health ally. A visit to the National Museum of Iceland (Þjóðminjasafn Íslands), websites such as www.syndum.is, or the bank of images provided by the University of Iceland attest to the documentation of water as a co-protagonist in the national narrative. The format and content of the visuals are in themselves evidence of how the island nation has redefined its relation to the ecosystem it inhabits. The introduction of technology to channel abundant geothermal resources marked the beginning of a new era in the country. It also reshaped the perception of what it means to heat homes with energy transported through tubes from sires connected to the subsurface of the Earth. In line with the main argument of the book, each society has its own interaction and dynamic with nature as a source of health and each component of nature occupies a place in the intimate imaginary of a society. Icelandic nature, distinguishable by glaciers, volcanoes, colorful lava fields with no trees, and surrounded by the cool temperatures of the North

Atlantic, shapes the life of its inhabitants and how they react to the ecosystem where they live.

The case of Iceland shows that water is linked to notions of staying healthy and of using the precious substance to stay disease free. By the same token, this places the same substance in a special place within the mindset of those that regard it as beneficial and important. In the context of bioclusivity, the intrinsic interdependence between humans and water in Iceland underpins an instinctive sense of symbiosis. This does not mean that the awareness about the use of natural resources is complete. Many people who have lived in Iceland, like the author of this book, have noticed, for instance, that in the swimming pool guests sometimes leave the shower running once they have completed their thorough pre-pool shower. A custom reinforced by shower guards, in case anyone misses the sign or is not familiar with this hygienical norm. The water runs, although now less so, since electric sensors have been introduced in some of the swimming pools across the country. While the unused water runs, visitors from countries with shortage of water fail to hide their bafflement and perplexity. Their expressions resemble the look on their faces when they follow the Icelandic procedure to get a glass of cold tap water. In order to avoid any mixture between the geothermally heated water (with a distinct smell and taste) and the bitterly cold water, Icelanders leave the tap open for a while. Personal experience and preference in terms of temperature (the longer, the colder the water gets) moderate how much unused water runs into the sink, again causing slight dismay among unaccustomed onlookers. "Why would you waste water like that?" I have heard from people asking Icelanders about their tap practices. The most common answer I can recall is that "if it runs it gets colder and tastes better and fresher." I argue that such an explanation emerges from a human-ecosystem link only those conversant in the codes of that specific place can understand. Icelanders manage, perceive, harness, and relate to water on their own terms. By the same token, they regard it as an element of their healthscapes.

Their distinct approach to water, and hence nature, does not mean Icelanders necessarily pollute less than other countries. On the contrary, judging from the numbers released in 2021, Iceland ranks high in per capita greenhouse gas emissions.[28] Compared to the small population, its footprint should be smaller, applying the envisioned goals applicable to advanced European economies. The images from the European agencies reporting on greenhouse gas emissions are visualizations in which each bar tells viewers/readers something about the fulfilled or non-fulfilled aspirations to build a Europe that pollutes less. They have an informational and inspirational side. They display what has been done and what needs to be done. Graphics and images characterize longing, desires, and ambitions, not only facts. Measurements indicate that Iceland's emissions per capita are disappointingly high—a constatation that cannot be negotiated. It is a fact. How Iceland, or other societies, relate to nature is, on the other hand, I argue, not an easy task to measure, and notwithstanding, it might hold the key to understanding the reasons and possible solutions to the future of the planet. Ultimately, planetarian balance will determine states of health and well-being at an individual level.

Representations (e.g., local horticultural products ad), at least partially, seem to provide a silhouette and a synopsis of the ontological underpinnings that define how collective imaginaries perceive nature. It seems that cultural expressions play a part in communicating attitudes about the relation between societies and topologies. The bioclusivity of each society may not be expressed entirely through the depiction of scientific data—even though science probably offers the most accurate information on how the natural world works—but it can nevertheless be seen through visual externalizations of the creating societies. Nature and health as theme and genre in visual culture reveal the sets of ideas cocooned in their materiality as cultural artifacts. From a reception standpoint, these images also play a role as they become vehicles to circulate ideas that, as this section shows, can prompt the adoption of practices, epistemic exchanges, or reconfiguration of attitudes. Bioclusivity is embedded in codes that have a high level of plasticity. Additions in knowledge systems, technological/ideological cross-fertilization, and adoption of ideas mobilized by close or distant societies can inform and reshape the interaction between communities, their habitats, and healthscapes. As I show in the next section of the chapter, just as in the case of Iceland (macro-level), external stimuli modify bioclusivity codes at a micro-level as well.

SPACES OF SELF-DISCOVERY AND MEDICINE

A hip-level shot of a patient lying on what looks like a medical linear accelerator and a zoomed-in heated stone held by a healer are the opening scenes of *Spirit Doctors* (2005), a documentary about Okanagan medicine and identity in the context of modern Canada. The 40-minute documentary, directed by Marie Burke, follows the journeys of self-discovery of the Cree/Dene-European filmmaker, soundman Don Howell, and a couple of Syilx/Okanagan healers Mary and Ed Louie.[29] The location is essential to understand the messages shared by Mary, the central figure of the documentary. Places are sources of healing if one knows where to look, as she implies. Geographical landscapes, such as the Similkameen Valley where the couple of Indigenous healers live, have the potentiality to become medicinal and curative sites. Mary explains that her main mission is to help a superior being, the Creator, in reaching out to those in need of help. The Okanagan healer makes no distinction between corporeal and spiritual disease and observes that aching bodies are in fact embodiments of souls that have forgotten to pay tribute to the ecosystems they inhabit.

A handful of moss (presumably, a *Racomitrium* species) Mary picks from the ground, as she asserts, is excellent to cure wounds. These small flowerless plants, as she sees them, are medicines provided by the Creator—one more example of the idea that healing nature surrounds us everywhere. By using the moss to cure someone, the tiny plant becomes part of the interaction between two living organisms, humans and plants. The exchange is an agreement and needs to take place in the context of respect between givers and receivers, she explains. Extracting from nature without responding in kind leads to unbalance. As she proceeds, it becomes clear that she regards herself as a part of a system that functions adequately only if all elements take responsibility for their part. Accountability starts with those practicing medicine and hence, Mary argues that

> when you work with people, there's a lot of the bad habits you need to let go. You can't go out drinking [pause] or taking drugs [pause] or sleeping with others. You can't do that, because you're an instrument that the spirits and the Creator work through to help their relatives and his children.

To a certain extent, Mary describes diseases as by-products of actions that have violated the codes that maintain a symbiotic system (*natura-Homo sapiens*) from collapsing. After working as a healer/medicine person for over 50 years, along with her husband, Ed, her main message is that the places we inhabit do not belong to us. Mary emphasizes on the fact that everything in nature is there to serve living organisms but that transgressing and dishonoring certain codes can bring along disastrous consequences. The main filming sites, the Louies's home in the Similkameen Valley and Spotted Lake (British Columbia), as Mary asserts, exemplify sites of connection between living beings and opportunities to observe Mother Earth's greatness and generosity.[30]

Spirit Doctors is evidence that there is a diversity of ways in which humans regard nature from a health viewpoint. Ed discusses dominant views on science and the position of Indigenous medicinal practices in twenty-first-century Canada (and perhaps most of the world). Mary speaks also openly about her peripheral position and how difficult it is to do a line of work that prevents her from charging for her services. Nevertheless, as she emphasizes, being a medicine woman is her call. It is also part of her legacy. After all, Mary is a direct descendant of her mentor (her own grandmother). In Mary's words, "I'd been with her since I was small, until she left me. So what she did every day, I saw and I heard, so that way, it was a natural way for me to grow up. It's a natural teaching." Okanagan beliefs are central in the documentary, having as subplot Mary's self-discovery journey. As she explains, she was hesitant to attend the call of becoming a healer and serving her community. At the same time, Burke hones on her own relation with her Indigenous ancestry, the ethical aspects of filming Aboriginal ceremonies, and the relation between media and cultures risking extinction. In her position as the main narrator, Burke delves into the problematic angle of using cinema as a tool to register Indigenous secret rituals.

In parallel, a third standpoint included in the documentary is the pathway that leads soundman Don Howell to rediscover a forgotten side of his identity and the duality of hybrid identities in countries with a history of colonization. As it appears, during filming, Howell receives the news that he has throat cancer. A revelation that, as he observes, leads him to complete perplexity. Like in Burke's case, the making of the film prompts him to question his identity and spiritual life. Howell's diagnosis and the context of the film urge him to take a position regarding his own attitudes toward healing, medicinal efficacy, and modernity vis-à-vis tradition. For viewers, suddenly, the opening scene makes sense. The images show Howell as he receives radiotherapy photon beams. The combination of a cutting-edge medicinal equipment, monitor units, and footage from a ritual indicates *Spirit Doctors* presents the stark contrast between approaches and techniques.

When discussing to which extent the camera documents Indigenous medicinal protocols, the filmmaker clarifies that the Louies along with a group of elders from other groups have the last word. Burke adds that only "they will decide what can be shown and what must remain locked in the spiritual world of mystery." Narcisse Blood (Blackfoot), Annie Parker (Shuswap), Jenny Cardinal (Cree), and Bert Crowfoot (Siksika) exchange thoughts with the director about the relationship between media, visual culture, and Indigenous cultural legacies. In the process, the documentary involves the audiences in a part of the process of creation of media artifacts not conventionally shown in indigeneity-oriented filmmaking, unless it is one of the main topics of the production. On this account, *Spirit Doctors* makes a statement about the role of agency in visual representation and self-representation. Beyond the pictorial value or illustrative qualities of images that communicate and inform, as Burke demonstrates, cultural expressions document and register worldviews, cosmologies, ontologies, and epistemic systems ingrained in each culture. Through narrative and cinematographic codes, angles, and takes, the film reiteratively insists on the gap between Aboriginal and mainstream Canadian (Western) medicine. It seems logical that the elders are involved in the transmission and circulation of images that touch upon intimate aspects of their epistemologies. The elders consulted agree on the fact that media can play a role in transmitting and rendering visible practices, sets of beliefs, and knowledge that would otherwise be lost. An observation that presumably applies, in particular, to communities living in contexts that challenge their survival as cultural entities.

Alternatively, the elders also express their concerns about the tendency to simplify Indigenous cultures and presume their epistemic practices can easily be encapsulated in a couple of images. If sacred ceremonies can have beneficial therapeutical, curative, or palliative effects on the human body, it does not sound logical, in the words of the elders, to assume their expertise is an easily transferable entity. By asking for consent and engaging in a conversation about the role of media in contemporary societies, Burke puts emphasis on the value of the knowledge being shared. Visual culture revolves around the production of images that disseminate various types of information through different pictorial formats. And semiotic codes. There is a distinction between form and content. In particular if one uses space as a frame of reference. The form (e.g., a video) might not be recognized as a valid vehicle to convey intimate details of healing rituals. As two of the elders observe, it is not the place for it. In fact, their remarks prompt the reflection that the only space in which the ceremonies are supposed to occur is in the designated sites, moments, and witnessed by those allowed to do so. The content (i.e., Indigenous medicine healing rituals) remains, as two of the elders postulate, outside the realm encompassed by images. From a bioclusivity perspective, these remarks reinforce the argument that each culture has its own understanding of nature and its own ways of expressing its relationship with it. The elders acknowledge the power of media as broadcasting, promulgation, and documentation tools. Yet, they reserve the sacredness of their beliefs to a place and time that escapes the lens of a camera. As Jenny Cardinal (Cree) explains, "Putting it on, on TV is a no no for me." Indigenous healthscapes follow protocols that are meant to unfold in allocated surroundings.

In this sense, there are three notions of topologies in *Spirit Doctors.* First, the sites in which ceremonies, rituals, and daily life take place and which include not only sacred territories (e.g., Spotted Lake, figure 5.2) but also modern-day facilities that signal the contrast between non-Indigenous and Indigenous lifestyles (e.g., the drugstore where Howell collects his medicines or the cancer treatment center where he receives radiotherapy). Second, the spiritual world that is not displayed through images but through the accounts and descriptions (oral tradition) of the Indigenous healers. As the film progresses, the spiritual realm becomes more present through the visual absence of the intangible territory in which, according to Mary, healing actually happens. Third, the camera that audiences cannot see either but that is also present and which records its own existence by the images it registers. *Spirit Doctors* is a recollection of visuals that lodge three parallel processes of transformation. The documentary follows the self-discovery journey of Burke as a filmmaker trusted by Mary to deliver a message that helps those in need.

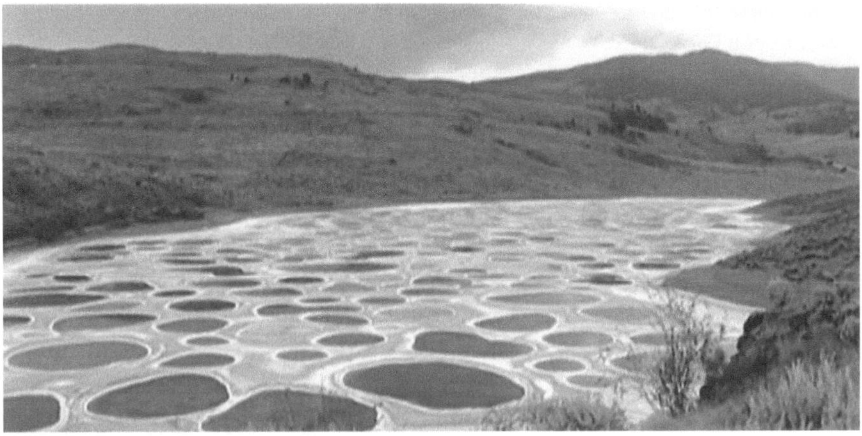

Figure 5.2 Screenshot from *Spirit Doctors* (2005).

Meanwhile, the filmmaker learns about the ethical protocols observed by a community to which she is related.

The film also sheds light on the culturally disruptive power of encounters between Aboriginal and Western epistemic practices, best exemplified by Howell's views on his own cancer treatment. After being treated by Mary, he expresses gratitude about finding his way back into an unattended facet of his life. Howell concludes that

> this is not, not *the* miracle cure. I don't believe this is *the* miracle cure. I believe this is only a part of the beginning. I definitely have a deeper understanding where my role is . . . um . . . in my healing now.

Burke and Howell seem to experience a change in their outlook toward who they are and what their role is. The circle closes. Their insights remind viewers of Mary's reflection on listening to her ancestors' call to become a medicine woman a year after the death of her son. As the title indicates, *Spirit Doctors* devotes a large part of the narrative to the centrality of spirituality as a legitimate element within the promotion of health and prevention of diseases.

It does not go unnoticed that the documentary seeks to draw attention to Mary's teachings. Water, in particular, receives special attention. As Mary explains, people in need of guidance and support can

> go to the water and ask it to help you get into it. Face the flow of it and help you to take the negativity away, the hurts, the pains. Go to the water as often as possible. If you can't go to the water then after your shower, shut off the hot water, and let the cold water hit you, because your, your spirit, still cries for the

> cold water for the strength that it needs to help you achieve your goals that is before you [*sic*].

It is essential that water remains clean because it is the blood running through the veins of Mother Earth, Mary adds. In the vicinity of the water, Herman Edwards, one of Mary's spiritual brothers, shares his views about the predominant form of disseminating knowledge in the twenty-first century. "And then today, if we don't read it in a book or in a paper, it don't mean nothing, people don't believe in things that are verbal [*sic*]," he says. *Spirit Doctors* highlights the perceived hierarchical system in which Indigenous medicine operates in a subaltern position compared to biomedicine. Edwards's remarks acquire a dramatic tone when he adds that Indigenous cultures might one day be "only memories." As Mary, he seems to participate in the creation of a portrait of their medicinal practices and shares his thoughts with Burke, emphasizing that health and nature are embedded in the same system. Taking care of the natural world is being conscious of the health of all living organisms.

The protocols that Mary and her spiritual fellows observe are part of a cultural and epistemic system that includes those who are conversant in them. Mary's vocabularies to describe the intertwined nature-health dyad, most likely, escapes or does not reach those who are not familiar with Okanagan culture. Clusivity, as a term derived from linguistics, can be useful to understand the proclivities and characteristics of systems that make distinctions between included and excluded sets of elements, beliefs, concepts, approaches, attitudes, and practices. Through her narrations, Mary attempts to chart an imaginary map for audiences to be able to navigate the topologies of her culture. Ed warns about the dangers they face when others mock them on the basis of their occupation as Indigenous medicine people. He admits not everyone is able or willing to recognize his approach to therapeutical, curative, and medicinal practices. Reiteratively, I suggest that it is through the presence and absence of codes, protocols, and epistemic practices, either derived from experience, observation, or rigorous examination, that each society adheres to its sense of bioclusivity.

Without seeking to question Okanagan medicine, I consult the protocols that I am trained to consider verifiable points of references, according to the ontological apparatus that has informed my worldviews. For me, my protocols reside in the production of knowledge that results from what I consider verified sources, use of the scientific method, experimentation, collection of data, and careful analysis. A tradition built on the notion that science emerges from (ideally) unbiased meticulous approaches, verifiable and replaceable, or corrected if they are not deemed to be reproducible or universal. Modern science documents findings in papers and books, as observed by Edwards, and those are the places where I search for any connection to Mary's epistemic practices.[31] I focus specifically on two aspects. The first one is the above-mentioned benefits of a species of *Racomitrium* mosses to alleviate injuries on the skin and the second one is the potential of exposure to cold water for improved mental and emotional well-being.

For over a century, scientists in various fields have studied the benefits and countereffects of cold water.[32] There is no definite conclusion to the matter, but increasing evidence shows it can prove beneficial for human health.[33] Studies confirm immersion in cold water can have long-term therapeutical applications. Some downsides include the instant psychological shock effect of overexposure to cold water for those who are not used to it. A body of scientific knowledge exists on the subject, also in terms of effect on the psychological and mental state of those, either swimming or immersing themselves in cold baths.[34] As for the mosses, they belong to the proposed taxonomic division of bryophytes, along with liverworts and hornworts. In some studies, they tend to be studied collectively and are somehow less understood than other plants endemic to so many parts of the globe. In general terms, their place in ethnological and cultural repertoire is relatively well documented and some medicinal benefits have been identified. While some studies indicate more research is needed,in others, the overall positive effects are salient (e.g., antimicrobial and antioxidant)—the main conclusion is that mosses can also cause allergies and some type of dermatitis.[35]

To clarify, this consultation of science-driven research is by no means intended to compare, contrast or falsify Mary's medicinal practices. The purpose is to establish a hypothetical dialogue between biomedicine and Okanagan medicine. Perhaps, a conversation that does not routinely takes place due to the hierarchy in which epistemic practices occur. Burke's documentary sheds light on the stark contrast between mainstream Canadian and Okanagan healthscapes. The elders, in all their right, are protective and custodial of their legacy, heritage, and ceremonies. The camera remains outside, in a place where it can freeze this knowledge in time and space, archive it, or accumulate it. The elders resist that idea and ethics primes over the need to create an artifact of self-expression. On the grounds of accountability, I ask myself if I am allowed to watch the documentary and eventually submit its content to a process of transcription and transposition in the form of these paragraphs. Through this text and perhaps others, Mary's teachings infiltrate (or are absorbed into) the written world. By extension, they enter the vortexes of information which are all part of larger editorial processes.

As opposed to the oral tradition celebrated and recognized by the Okanagans, graphically documented material risks exposing the circulated content to eventual processes of decontextualization, framing, and decentering. Even if succinctly, this book registers nevertheless in paper pieces of knowledge shared by Mary orally. Medicine seems to be linked to epistemic regimes that are not meant to change or be easily overruled. Alternatively, reflecting on the place of *Spirit Doctors*, within the visualization of Indigenous protocols, one can conclude that both traditions observe well-determined conventions. Like texts, images, in general, registered by a camera are reportorial, editable, and configurable according to the author's subjectivity, to a large extent. On the documentation aspects of culture that are not intended to be expressed pictorially, one of the elders consulted, Narcisse Blood (academic, ceremonialist, filmmaker, educator), notes that

> when you don't know who you are, *ksaahkomm*, Mother Earth, will have trouble recognizing you. That's the way we see. Now, that's an aspect of our ceremonies that becomes a whole different worldview of experience, of experiencing that—these equipment, this modern day could be used as a tool in our favor, but it could never, ever replace that experience [*sic*].

Blood's insights underline how the particularities of each culture denote its relationship with the care and cure of their bodies and the spaces they occupy, either as individuals or as parts of communities. At a macro-level, an example of which is the abovementioned Icelandic outdoor bathing tradition, or at a micro-level, typified by Mary's daily activities as Indigenous medicine woman, humans engage in health-enhancing practices. Their sense of how nature plays a role in their worldviews, or what I call bioclusivity, defines also in which way their habitats become part of their pursuit to stay disease free and live well. The topologies of health are the sites humans believe can activate their capacity to achieve what they imagine or conceive as healthiness. Scientific research provides one the most accurate pictures of how the natural world operates but not necessarily an image of how *natura-Homo sapiens* dynamic culturally unfolds. Visuals offer insights into cultural practices not commonly found in other forms of documentation. The tridimensionality of healthscapes embowers the tripartite dimension explored in this book, health-nature-images, showing that epistemic health practices are part of the bioclusivity spectrum of each society.

NOTES

1. Madan (2019).
2. Cox (2013); Seelig (2019).
3. It is important to note that ecological understandings have found their way into pictorial representations even before there was a sense of consensus and awareness about the implications of human-induced climatic change. Concerns about ecosystems and human impact on them are themes that can be identified in

nineteenth-century visual culture (Coughlin and Gephart, 2020). Media as health-promoting spaces are not new either. Mass health campaigns are at least four decades old (Randolph and Viswanath, 2004). Recent developments include specifically a focus on sustainability (Barkemeyer, Givry and Figge, 2018), and the effects of industrialization on climatic change (Sklair, 2020). Conceptually, Mirzoeff (2009, 2014) suggests that visualizing ecological unbalance requires noticing the historical implications in the creation of pictorial representations, placing emphasis on how images chronicle processes, hegemonic attitudes, and invisibility of less powerful segments of the world population.

4. Monani and Adamson (2017).

5. Friðjónsdóttir (2020). About the expression, it is a colloquialism used to describe an event, situation, or state that causes sorrow and sadness.

6. Jónsson (2013).

7. Before harnessing geothermal energy became a nationwide project, the first experiments to pipe hot water for domestic use were carried out in the form of home-made experiments in farms around the country, among others, by Stefáns B. Jónssonar, Erlendur á Sturlureykjum, and Sigurjóns á Álafossi (Þórðarson, 1998).

8. Þórðarson (1998).

9. Einarsson (1945) also notes although the number of swimmers in Iceland had dropped dramatically throughout the ages, records attest the existence of "góðir sundmenn" (good swimmers) (2) since the Age of Settlement.

10. Estimates indicate that around 4,000 Icelanders drowned in the twentieth century (Bjarnason, 2017).

11. Einarsson (1945).

12. *Norðanfari* (1875), *Ísafold* (1889), *Þjóðviljinn* (1891).

13. Pétursson (1989).

14. The manual built on instructional material written by Franz Nachtegall (1777–1847), one of Denmark's early proponents of teaching gymnastics and physical education as part of school curricula.

15. Sport Law decree 517/557 approved in 1940 stipulates that all children in the country, unless exempt for medical reasons, should receive swimming lessons and be able to swim before they turn 14 (Alþingi, 1940, art. 13). Since its introduction as in the Icelandic school system, *sund* has had for a special status as, in principle, students cannot successfully finish their education without knowing how to swim. Professional specialized teachers oversee that the training includes the practicalities of the main styles, strokes, and techniques.

16. Findings from recent scholarly work on the history of TB in Iceland indicates that the disease was introduced in the country much earlier. In a paleontological study, 274 skeletons extracted from Hofstaðir, Keldudalur, and Skeljastaðir were examined for signs of disease. In total, tuberculosis-related lesions were found in 32 of them. Pott's diseases, lymphadenitis, and iliopsoas abscesses are some of the other diseases identified in the skeletons. Conclusively, findings from this study indicate the presence of tuberculosis in Iceland soon after the first settlers took up residence on the island nation. Presumably, by late tenth and mid-thirteenth century, the disease became endemic in certain parts of the country (Collins, 2020).

17. Sigurðsson (1976) notes that between 1920s and 1930s, tuberculosis was the main cause of death in 20% of the cases, despite government's efforts to combat the disease, for instance, by allocating around 8% of the national budget to TB-related costs.

18. Original text in Icelandic: "í sambandi við aukna líkamsræktun þjóðarinnar, er lífsnauðsyn að upp rísi, jafnt í sveitinni sem bæjum, baðstofur, þar sem gufuböð yrðu stunduð af öllum almenningi, eins og hér tíðkaðist á landnámsöld. Mestu heilbrigðisérfræðingar og íþróttafrömuðir nútímans, hafa komizt að þeirri niðurstöðu eftir ýtarlegar rannsóknir, að hin einfalda gamla finsk-rússneska baðstofa, sem notuð hefir verið í þessum tveim löndum í þúsund ár, sé sá lífsaflgjafi er nútíma menningin verði að tileinka sér. Frændur vorir, Svíar, sem taldir eru standa framarlega sem menningarþjóð, eru nú í þann veginn, að breyta stærstu baðstöðum sínum þannig, að þeir samrýma þá þúsund ára reynslu finsk-rússnesku baðstofunnar " (Kuld, 1939, 2).

19. Original text in Icelandic: "— Hvers vegna fórstu að iðka þessi hlaup um bæinn?— Ætli það hafi ekki verið fyrir áhrif frá dr. Helga Pjeturss. Hann hljóp manna mest um bæinn sér til heilsubótar og var æði vígalegur, stundum, þegar hann hljóp með lyftingartæki á lofti í hvorri hendi. En þessar göngur, hlaup og útivist voru máske heist sprottnar af ótta við tæringuna, sem þá fór hér um eins og eldur í sinu. En margir töldu það ráð gegn berklunum að vera sem mest á hreyfingu úti við, iðka sund og hlaup. Það gerði dr. Helgi Pjeturss í áratugi, gekk og hljóp i sjóinn eða sundlaugarnar á hverjum drottins degi og stældi skrokkinn, enda bar hann sig vel fram á elliár" (Bergmann, 1964: 8).

20. See, for instance, *Heilbrigðistíðindi* (issued on June 1, 1879), *Eimreiðin* (May 1, 1914), *Ísafold* (April 7, 1927), and "Finsk baðstofa tekur öllum böðum fram" (Einarsson, 1938).

21. Baggio, Qadir and Smakhtin (2021).

22. Studies on the quality of Icelandic water do confirm that "the chemical quality of drinking water is generally good in Iceland with only a few incidents of noncompliance with regulations, mostly as regards indicators or aesthetic parameters. Compliance of Icelandic drinking water with chemical quality is over 99% which is among the highest in the 28 member states of the European Union' (Gunnarsdóttir, Garðarsson, Jónsson and Bartram, 2016, 732).

23. Samtök iðnaðarins (Federation of Icelandic Industries) proposed in 2013 to change the law pertaining the use of the national flag as a labeling strategy to specify in which cases a product can be considered to be Icelandic (Neytendablaðið, 2013). According to the current regulations, if a vegetable or fruit for sale is not farmed in Iceland, the use of the flag is forbidden.

24. As I suggest in other chapters, this combination of images and text are examples of pictograph-ness.

25. Jóhannesson (2010).

26. The ads appeared in *Fréttablaðið*, *Morgunblaðið*, and *Skessuhorn* between May and August 2018.

27. Hastrup (2008) suggests that the idea of purism in Iceland might be linked to the notion of timelessness.

28. Clarke, Heinonen and Ottelin (2017).

29. Okanagan is a cover designation for many subgroups encompassed in the Indigenous term used for a linguistic continuum (*nsilxcín*) and an anglicization of *ukwnaqínx*. For more information, see the website of The Yinka Déné Language Institute.

30. Roed and Fulton (2011) observe that the lake has had a special place as a revered site for centuries due to the presumed therapeutic properties of its water.

31. Although any comparison of this kind builds on premises that are not necessarily analog. Focusing on the case of Tibetan medicine, Adams (2001) reminds us that debates about efficacy of medicinal practices that involve a spiritual component are "not simply about naming; they are rather about what the debate over naming can tell us about the meaning of 'science' through its uses *as a signifier* in this locale" (570).

32. Some of the studies carried out in the twentieth century include work done by James Currie (1804), Edgar Hines and George Brown (1932), David Clarke (1963), George Stelmach (with Clarke) (1966), and Mike Tipton (1989). In the third decade of the nineteenth century, Vincenz Prießnitz (1799–1851) played an important role in reviving the use of hydrotherapeutic techniques, first in the German-speaking world and then further afield in Europe. Prießnitz's work seems to have inspired Sebastian Kneipp (1821–1897) in the development of a set of therapies (Kneippism) that involved the use of cold water (Kirchfeld and Boyle, 1994). Prießnitz and Kneipp's approaches were adopted in several spa facilities throughout Europe (Baumgarten, 2015). However, they remained highly controversial for being considered unscientific alternative medicine, although followed and praised by practicing physicians as well (Andresen, 1875).

33. The literature on this is substantial, but studies by LaFoy and Geden (1989), Huttunen (2004), Shevchuk and Radoja (2007), Silva et al. (2008), Khaltaev et al. (2020), Bekiari et al. (2021), and Fujita et al. (2022) show the empirically tested applicability of water for therapeutic purposes.

34. Swift (1932); LeBlanc et al. (1960); Livingstone et al. (1978); Ishikawa et al. (1992); Kenny et al. (1999); Rasmussen and Mercer (2004) ; Mantoni et al. (2007) ; Solianik et al. (2014) ; Muzik et al. (2017) ; Heinonen et al. (2018) ; Hohenauer et al. (2019) ; Knechtle (2020).

35. See Marko et al. (2001); Harris (2008); Sabovljević (2016); Horn et al. (2021); Wolski et al. (2021).

Chapter 6

Sensorial Interfaces

Nobody seems immune to the effect of psychoactive substances once they come in contact with the body to which it belongs. That is a fact well known by the tourists making their way into any of the *coffeeshops/koffieshops* in Amsterdam or any customer entering one of the Uruguayan *farmacias* (pharmacies) selling alpha- and beta-type bags of cannabis. The visuality of soft drugs in The Netherlands materializes mostly through leaf-decorated souvenirs (e.g., lighters and ashtrays) (figure 6.1) and creative signs of cannabis-selling establishments and in Uruguay through awareness campaigns (e.g., a post of a scissor tracing a line between marihuana and a pregnant woman).[1] One element, or rather, one place, is commonly missing in the visual representation of references surrounding psychoactive substances, and for obvious reasons, the human mind. Psychotropics scape the categorical definition of health as the state of being free of disease or injury. At least, in principle, and except in case of overconsumption and abuse, allegedly, they do not cause sickness or physically harm or hurt recreational users.

Addiction and misuse are major issues, nevertheless. In fact, addiction has the potential of becoming a biopsychosocial compulsiveness-driven disorder with devastating consequences for those who suffer from it, many of whom never recover or learn to manage it. Psychotropics have an impact on our brain and nervous systems, eventually manifesting in behaviors and perception. The list of side effects of psychoactive substances from a clinical standpoint explains, to a large extent, their history from a sociocultural perspective, even if psychotropic substances have accompanied humanity for millenniums.[2] Today, in most countries across the globe, there are more or less certain regulations about their use, cultivation, preparation, circulation, and commercialization.[3] Networks implemented to smuggle them have emerged hand in hand with high levels of criminality, violence, impunity,

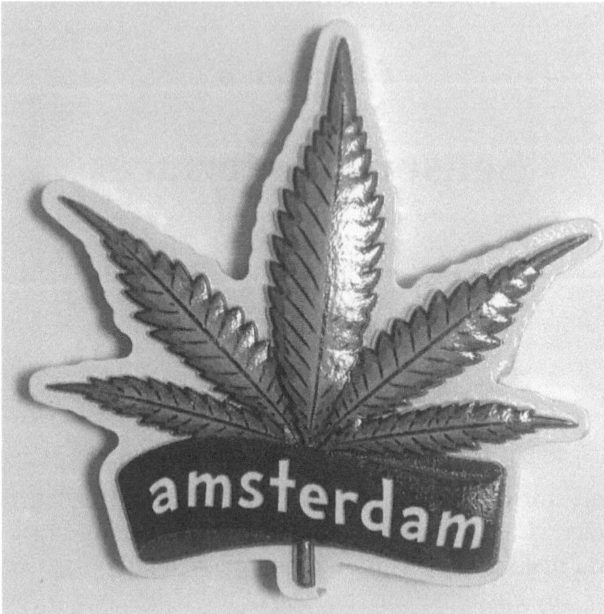

Figure 6.1 Cannabis Souvenir. *Source*: Photo by author.

and corruption. The appetite for mind-altering recreational substances has destroyed not only many consumers but also the social fabric of the countries where raw materials grow or where labs operate, with some exceptions.[4] Some are naturally farmed and some are chemically produced. Psychoactive agents are present in, for instance, mushrooms, flowers, cacti, lianas, and leaves. Advances in modern chemistry have allowed for the development and mass production of substances that, mostly illegally, supply the global high demand for, what many colloquially call simply *drugs*.

Addiction, dependence, misuse, and the social implications thereof have ignited a war against recreational substances, fought on many fronts, and, yet, unsuccessful in many respects. Health is the raison d'être behind the majority of antidrug campaigns, legal implementations, judicial frameworks, and collaborative efforts to prevent the use of psychotropics. Production and supply, as stipulated in the *Single Convention on Narcotic Drugs* (1961), have resulted in a relatively well-demarcated line that positions psychoactive agents, according to certain contexts, at either side of a well-demarcated line between licit and illicit. Special licenses apply to medicinal use, for instance, as part of spiritual and religious rituals and scientific research. These special provisions make concessions about their use as entheogens, not only acknowledging that psychotropics have a cultural dimension but also making a distinction between recreation, rituality, cosmovision, and tradition.

Entheogens are psychoactive substances inscribed in spiritual, religious, or ancestral practices and ritualized contexts, most of which, commonly but not necessarily, are derived from plant sources, but due to advances in chemistry, chemically synthesized entheogens do exist. In different parts of the world, psychotropics play a role as vehicles to engage in sacred events or to induce ceremonial trances, closer to meditation than to leisure or entertainment. In this sense, entheogenic use of psychoactive agents remains within the bioclusivity canons of societies for whom these substances operate as natural catalyzers of specific states of mind. Applying knowledge about the universality of the human body means that psychotropics affect everyone's mind in one way or another, whether this happens in recreational or spiritual settings. Or that was at least the logic applied by those who brought, for instance, peyote and San Pedro cacti to American and European labs, inducing the birth of a line of pharmaceuticals that after a decade-long hiatus, might be about to come back. A Psychedelics Renaissance in which psychotropics revolutionize mental health pharmacology is, according to some, already in the making.[5] The history of mind-altering substances is, from many perspectives, the chronicle of encounters, mobilization of natural resources, bodily practices, secrecy, allure, and curiosity. Visual media have recorded this trajectory, as a story marked by exchanges and shifts where the human mind is the only constant and yet invisible element.

HALLUCINATORY TRANSMOGRIFICATION

Images and written texts of various types, mobilized across Western Europe during the twentieth century, have circulated ideas about the medicinal properties of entheogens originated from the Americas. The promotion, circulation, and commercialization of entheogens have been reshaped by unequal epistemic and material exchanges, stereotypical paradigms, and schemas embedded in Eurocentric imaginaries about the positionality of Indigenous peoples. Part of a process Boumediene (2016) calls *la colonisation du savoir* (the colonization of knowledge). Amerindian entheogens in Western labs and their eventual synthesization enact the materiality of knowledge transfers and additions at a transatlantic level, and by proxy, they are evidence of the epistemic presence of societies, often considered as peripheral, from the perspective of institutionalized formal circles of knowledge production. If we are indeed at the beginning of a psychedelic renaissance, as the present has been described by many in terms of neuroscientific advances and possible capitalization, for instance, of ayahuasca derivatives, it matters to understand in which ways beliefs have defined, conditioned, and disciplined previous materia medica exchanges involving mind-altering substances.[6]

If we all dwell within the borders of our own bioclusivity, this position presumably involves a set of specific bodies of knowledge that reflect the ecosystems we call home. From that perspective, epistemic extraction occurs as much as a natural resource extraction occurs. Synthesized entheogens show the transmogrifying processes involved in the circulation of natural precursors across different systems, epistemologies, ontological orders, and epistemic practices. Plants (or other living organisms) traditionally used in ritualistic settings logically acquire a different meaning in the backdrop of a laboratory. Entheogen as a term that distinguishes between recreational and cultural substances indicates we are aware of the bioclusivity paradigms that define our relation to the natural world. Legal definitions emerge precisely to mark categorizations that set boundaries and emphasize margins. It is not the morphology of mind-altering substances that determines their stratification within the various systems in which they circulate, but the cultural (and by extension legal, political, socioeconomic, biosocial, medical) criteria at play. Its non-pharmaceutically, but culturally, determined connotation is central to understanding the various roles and meanings of entheogens in different settings and for a diverse array of purposes. In the next paragraphs, the main focus lies on reviewing the visual and textual framing of *Lophophora williamsii* (i.e., peyote), Psilocybin mushrooms (e.g., *Psilocybe mexicana*), and, briefly, brews produced of mixing *Banisteriopsis caapi* and *Psychotria viridis* (i.e., ayahuasca).

First reported by Spanish friars during the colonization of the Americas, entheogens from the New World have been socially conditioned by religious ideas about conscious-altering properties, legal constraints imposed on psychoactive substances, and scientific enterprises to isolate, synthesize, and harness their possible applications. Examples of natural, mind-altering precursors that have retained a sense of exceptionality conferred by their use by legally acknowledged Indigenous communities include peyote, sacred datura, and ayahuasca brews.

From the first encounters between Europeans and pre-Columbian peoples in the late fifteenth century, images and written texts have recorded the use of plants to induce psychoactive states with profound effects on the human mind (e.g., hallucinations) and human body (e.g., severe nausea and vomiting). They were described as part of practices informed by medicinal, spiritual, and social protocols inflected by a wide understanding that these substances could be not only beneficial but also harmful.[7] The institution of the Spanish Inquisition, moved by religious agenda, disapproved strongly the use of mind-altering drugs among Indigenous populations. Notwithstanding, members of the Catholic church were among the first to document and describe the effect of psychoactive substances and their centrality within spiritual and ceremonial settings.

Equating hallucinations with (dark) magic was the beginning of the prohibitive approach applied to these substances during the Colonial period. In his multivolume ethnographic project *La Historia General de las Cosas de Nueva España/The Universal History of the Things* of *New Spain*, Bernardino de Sahagún wrote on the subject:

> Its leaves are slender, cord-like, small. Its name is ololiuhqui. It makes one besotted; it deranges one, troubles one, maddens one, makes one possessed. He who eats it, who drinks it, sees many things which greatly terrify him. He is really frightened [by the] poisonous serpent which he sees for that reason. He who hates people causes on to swallow it in drink [and] food to madden him.[8]

Ololiuhqui (figure 6.2) has been identified as Christmas vine/Morning Glory (*Ipomoea corymbosa/Turbina corymbosa*, Granziera, 2001).[9] Images of the plant ornamenting Sahagún's unique book are among the first sites of visual mediation of psychoactive precursors from the Americas.

In the 11th book of this work, commonly known as the Florentine Codex, and the product of a collaboration between the Nahua people and Sahagún, five entheogens are mentioned. On *Peiotl*, the text in Nahuatl states that

> this peyote is white and grows only in the north region called Mictlan. On him who eats it or drinks it, it takes effect like mushrooms. Also he sees many things which frighten one, or make one laugh. It affects him perhaps one day, perhaps

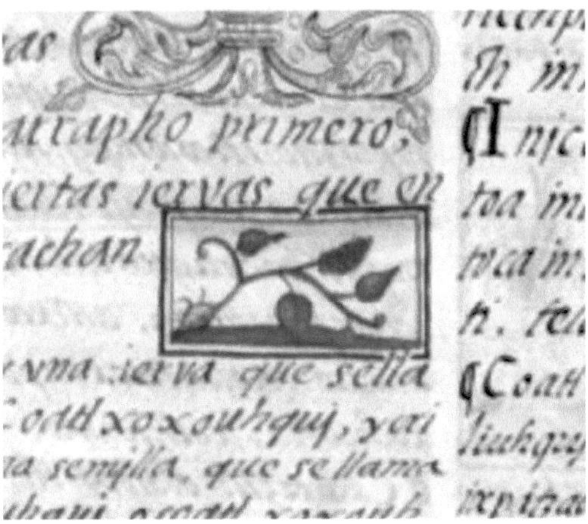

Figure 6.2 Drawing of *ololiuhqui*, Ornamenting a Paragraph on Psychotropics in *La Historia General de las Cosas de Nueva España*, Folio 129, Book X1, Volume 7 (1545–1590). *Source*: Courtesy of World Digital Library.

> two days, but likewise it abates. However, it harms one, troubles one, makes one besotted, takes effect on one. I take peyote; I am troubled.[10]

Despite its side effects, peyote remained nevertheless attractive to the Spanish citizens living in the Viceroyalty of New Spain (present-day Mexico) because of its presumed divinatory faculties. To the extent that its use became illicit in 1620.[11] These warnings did not intimidate inquisitive colonizers, traders, explorers, and scholars, either in the decades that followed after the first encounters between pre-Columbian nations and Europeans or in the centuries thereafter. In contrast with the traditional role of psychoactive agents (e.g., premonitory, and therapeutic), their recreational use have always reflected an appetite for altered states of consciousness. Mind-altering precursors allure also those interested in their commercialization and possible applications. Chemists and pharmacologists have not only toyed with but also seriously explored ways to adapt entheogens into pharmaceutical derivatives and therapeutic agents. During the early and mid-twentieth century, scientific endeavors lead to more understanding about the pharmacology of their components. Moved by the inquisitiveness of his brother's adventures in Mexico, John Raleigh Briggs (1851–1907), a doctor and medical journal editor based in Fort Worth (Texas), was the first one to describe scientifically his own experience after ingesting peyote buttons in 1886. An experience he shared publicly in *The Medical Bulletin* with these words:

> At 10 a.m., June 20, 1886, I ate one-third of one of those "buttons," or prickly plants and with pencil and paper and watch before me, awaited results. In fifteen minutes afterward I felt a slight fulness in my carotids, and found my pulse had gone from 60 normal to 70. In fifteen minutes more the feeling in my head and throat was becoming very unpleasant—one of over-arterial tension—and my pulse had reached 90. My respirations had gone up to this time from 18 normal to 26. The unpleasant fulness of my head rapidly increased until 10:45, when my head began to ache and I felt dizzy. My pulse had then reached 120 and respirations 30. Soon after the forty-five minutes had passed a sudden and alarming jump in my pulse occurred—reaching 160. The peculiar and dazed feelings I then experienced, together with alarm, prevented my taking notes on respirations, and therefore don't know the number, but they had certainly still further increased. It seemed to me my heart was simply running away with itself, and it was with considerable difficulty I could breathe air enough to keep me alive. I felt intoxicated, and for a short time particularly lost consciousness. (Briggs, 1887, 145)

In his note on his self-experimentation test, the Texan physician explains that *muscale buttons*, as peyote was also known, induce hallucinations that "those superstitious Indians" (145) perceive as reality and as part of their spiritual and religious practices. The visions, he proceeds as he questions them, apparently quoting an informant, include "'buffalo and wild horses come up out of the earth'(?)" (144). There was nothing ceremonial or recreational in Briggs's experiment, but the medical community took note.[12] Seven years later, Parke-Davis pharmaceuticals, owned by Pfizer today, and known for marketing medicines derived from expeditions to the tropics (e.g., Cascara-based laxatives), launched peyote tinctures to be used for heart and breathing-related conditions. While experiments with peyote in America as a potential natural precursor of pharmaceuticals to treat mental diseases failed, the plant kept circulating across European labs.

In 1918, Ernst Späth succeeded in synthesizing mescaline, the natural psychedelic alkaloid found in peyote and other cacti.[13] The synthesization of lysergic acid diethylamide (LSD) by Albert Hoffman in 1938 eclipsed in certain ways the development of a mescaline niche culture, although not entirely. Mescaline drew circles of artists, intellectuals, and bohemians, seduced by the stimuli mescaline allegedly had on human creativity and willingness to experiment with it. By the 1930s, inquiries into the pharmacology and effects of mescaline by scientists and psychiatrists had already not only been registered in scholarly publications but had also tacitly been registered in works of art. Surrealist painters such as Stanisław Ignacy Witkiewicz is known for agreeing to participate in such experiments.[14] Artists would consume mescaline and depict their visions on a canvas. Besides Witkiekicz's works (e.g., *Portrait of Stefan Glass*, 1929), the visuality of compounds derived from natural psychoactive cacti is solidified, for instance, in paintings by Julian Trevelyan (e.g., *Kites and Shapes*, 1936) and Herbrand Williams (e.g., *Mescaline*, 1936). The synthesization of mescaline was gradual, inspiring, and informing at each step of the mobilization of ideas about its possible applications.

Indigenous knowledge(s) and cultural references served to contextualize, explain, and, in some ways, legitimize innovations. From the 1930s, advertisements for an innovative product started to appear in major newspapers in France, sometimes accompanied by drawings of cacti.[15] The texts vary, but the main message in them is that extract from peyote cactus can cure phobias and make those taking the round-shaped pills become more social. Peyote Tramni, as the product is called, also helps with *la maladie du scrupule*, a condition originally conceptualized by medieval theologists, not doctors, overlapping somehow with modern-day obsessive neurosis but mainly understood as the bodily reaction to Christian guilt and socially driven repentance.[16] The pills were briefly promoted as a panacea for mental conditions, ranging from depression to nervous breakdowns, tiredness, fears, undesired behavior, and moodiness. A medicine that cured bad mood, endorsed by the long experience of the Incas on the matter probably sounded tempting to many of the readers. The marketing strategy was indexical of the set of ideas about Mesoamerican civilizations and the dynamics of their knowledge(s):

foreign, alluring, and magical. Claims such as the regeneration of cells raise questions about the scientific rigor used by the laboratory behind the development and commercialization of the short-lived pharmacological formula. There seemed to be a widespread belief that Indigenous medicines might have benefits to trait conditions overlooked by biomedicine. Peyote Tramni is presented as an innovation derived from Mexican ancestral peoples and as a natural alternative for conditions not easily treatable with biochemicals. Since some of the advertisements mention the Inca civilization, a possible explanation is that the Paris-based laboratory had access to San Pedro *cactus* (*Trichocereus pachanoi*).

Two decades after being first identified and isolated by Arther Heffter, mescaline was quite present in experimental psychiatry and as a hallucinogen among European urban circles and elites. Media circulation of images played a central role in the dissemination of ideas about mescaline (e.g., Henri Michaux, Belgian-born painter, *Mescaline Drawing* 1960). Visual allusions to the substance were indirectly traces of the Indigenous epistemologies and epistemic systems. An aspect that is easily overlooked when reviewing the history of pre-Columbian *Peiotl* cactus derivatives outside Mesoamerica. By the time LSD became a recreational drug in the 1960s, mescaline had already left a dent in the way psychotropic substances were presented across media spaces. Reactions of audiences were divided into those negatively impacted by the idea of substances with consciousness-altering properties and those who celebrated the reverberations of counter-culture's impact on the social landscape. The human mind was present in public discourse not in the form of an image but as the main topic underlying the discussion about psychotropics.

Interest in psychoactive substances on both sides of the Atlantic encouraged the exploration of new frontier territories for science but older known realms for anthropologists and linguists. On June 29, 1955, Gordon Wasson and his wife, Valentina Pavlovna, visited María Sabina, a Mazatec *curandera* (healer) who introduced them into the world of *veladas* ceremonies. During these spiritual rites, *niños* mushrooms (as they were known) (e.g., *Psilocybe mexicana*) would be eaten. Mushrooms were used for healing and for interaction with the unknown. The article in the magazine *Life* (1957), followed by an avalanche of articles, recordings of her evocative song-poem chants, and appearance in CBS's widely popular program *Person to Person* encouraged many to visit María Sabina. It was the central piece in the highly influential American magazine that gave visibility to the story. Wasson provided Albert Hofmann with some samples that he eventually isolated in his lab in Switzerland in 1959. Isolation of psilocybin paved the road for the emergence of Indocybin—a pharmaceutical that was originally used for its benefits in the treatment of mental and psychological disorders, such as anxiety and depression. The global circulation networks used by Swiss pharmaceutical company

Sandoz expanded the geographical range of the medicine and its eventual use, for instance, in veterinary settings. Like peyote, *Psilocybe mexicana* had undergone a morphological change. They were not inducers of ceremonial trances or spiritual enhancers, but chemically produced compounds carefully packaged and shipped internationally.

Just as in the case of peyote, cultural expressions have served to register the role of *niños* as intimate aspects of Mazatec bioclusivity. The sounds of that evening in June in which María Sabina met with the Wasson's have registered (and recorded in cassettes) the religious aspect in which the ingestion of mushroom is inscribed. The translation of the lyrics evokes the Mazatec own adaptations of the long-standing syncretic praxis that have distinguished the mixture of Indigenous and Catholic belief systems. As Eunice Pike, a Mazatec language student who assisted the Wasson's with the translation of the song mentions, prompting and experiencing visions, becomes a matter of being conversant in the culture where the tradition emerged.[17] Knowledge about the pharmacodynamics of cacti plants reveals the accumulation of descriptive facts, procedures, and the interaction with instruments applied to interact with the objects believed to have therapeutic and medicinal properties.

Advances in Western laboratories and legal conventions molded by the interest of Western versus non-Western countries (e.g., Convention on Psychotropic Substances, 1971) has furthermore reshaped the accessibility, interest, circulation, and medicinal materiality of psychoactive substances ever since. Entheogens as substances used as medications to cure or alleviate symptoms have not officially entered or passed product approval thresholds. *Lophophora williamsii* (i.e., peyote), *Datura wrightii* (i.e., sacred datura), and brews produced by mixing *Banisteriopsis caapi* and *Psychotria viridis* (i.e. ayahuasca) have not yet materialized as medicines, at least not so far, even if "renaissance of psychedelic research" grows gradually and progressively.[18] To various extents, the circulation of entheogens through Western laboratories has been characterized by hypothesis, design, synthesis, and some form of preclinical and clinical research. In other cases, it has been a matter of inquiry into pharmacological properties, ethnobotanical diversity, or recollection of samples for archival purposes (figure 6.3).

From a scientific perspective, it is not relevant if they are originally natural precursors embedded in epistemologies where their use is not only medicinal but also spiritual, holistic, and religious. Objects travel across ontologies when they circulate cross-culturally. The epistemological and epistemic settings in which these biopsychosocial materia medica substances emerge cannot possibly be preserved through cultural, geographical, legal, commercial, and material adaptation processes. I argue that it is a matter of bioclusivity. Legally, substances used in religious praxis of the occult, such as divination (from Latin, "foreseeing," etymologically derived from *divinare*, "inspired by

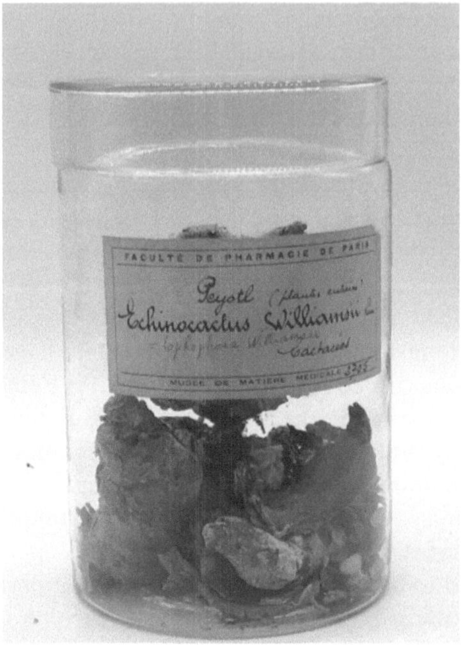

Figure 6.3 Peyotl (*Echinochactus williamsii*), Faculty of Pharmacy. *Source*: Courtesy of Musée François Tillequin, Paris Descartes University.

God"), were categorized according to the potential use authorities anticipated in contexts culturally dystonic with their origins. The journey of entheogens from the Americas in Western contexts mirror attempts to discipline the flux of knowledge while adapting it to localized sites and practices. Disciplining the mind is central in certain cultures, less so in others. Much has been written about the adoption, reception, and adaptation of Indigenous knowledge(s) in Western settings, nonetheless, in contexts of monetization and appropriation. María Sabina's observations about outsiders not "respecting" tradition hold from a spiritual and religious perspective. Nonetheless, materia medica transfers, as the ones I have explored in this section, demonstrate they are simultaneously epistemic additions. These transplants and the processes around them also demonstrate that biopsychosocial materia medica is understood differently according to the milieus in which it becomes instrumental for the societies interacting with it. Natural precursors mutate in the settings where they become part of the ecological, cultural, and social environment. An uprooted plant can be the beginning of a new chapter in the long durée history of the nature-health tandem.

TRANSPLANTED, DISCIPLINED, AND DE-STIGMATIZED

Originally endemic to Central and South Asia, cannabis (including both *Cannabis sativa* and *Cannabis indica*) has a long history as entheogen, medicine, forbidden drug, and allowed, within limits, recreation substances in places like Canada, Georgia, South Africa, Uruguay, and The Netherlands. Its effect on the human body and, in particular, on the human mind, has defined its long and tumultuous course across legal systems (crime), laboratories, and illicit production centers in all corners of the globe. Few plants elicit as much controversy, stir, debate, and tension. Few psychotropics have received as much visual and public space in cultural representations and media outlets.

Under different names, perhaps disguised by euphemisms, or in recent years, out in the open, cannabis is entering a phase of de-stigmatization. Or so it seems, based on the revisions that many countries are doing in their soft drug criminalization policies. The idea that the mind is a place to be disciplined by the state through the prohibition of psychoactive agents is rapidly mutating. Legalizing psychotropics is a revolutionary step, nonetheless, because of health concerns (e.g., addiction) and possible impact on younger generations. Canada, Georgia, Malta, Mexico, Portugal, South Africa, Uruguay, and a number of states in America have implemented and are implementing new approaches to the consumption of cannabis (either legalization or decriminalization). The Netherlands has had a policy, *gedoogbeleid* (policy of tolerance) since the 1990s. The government of the country explains its policy to the visitors of its official website in these terms:

> Toleration policy regarding soft drugs and coffee shops: Soft drugs are less damaging to health than hard drugs. In the Netherlands, coffee shops are permitted to sell cannabis under certain strict conditions. A coffee shop is an establishment where cannabis may be sold but no alcoholic drinks may be sold or consumed. This is part of the Dutch policy of toleration. Toleration policy regarding soft drugs: The Netherlands has a policy of toleration regarding soft drugs. This means that the sale of soft drugs in coffee shops is a criminal offence but the Public Prosecution Service does not prosecute coffee shops for this offence. Neither does the Public Prosecution Service prosecute members of the public for possession of small quantities of soft drugs. (Rijksoverheid, 2021)[19]

The rules about the quantities imply not having in one's possession more than 5 grams of cannabis, either marijuana (*wiet*) or hash (*hasj*) or the equivalent of 5 cannabis plants. Coffee shops (e.g., soft drug selling venues) must observe well-stipulated rules, such as not selling hard drugs, having customers who are underage, and surpassing the permitted quantities in one transaction. In an attempt to prevent drug tourism, since January 1, 2013, the government wants coffee shops to “focus on the local market.”[20] In theory, this means that soft drugs are only to be sold to *ingezetenen van Nederland* (residents of The Netherlands). This is (in theory) the end of the “open-door policy” and one of the many strategies implemented by Dutch municipalities, in particular, in large and border cities and towns, to combat the implications of *gedoogbeleid*. However, as any citizen of Amsterdam would agree, it is obvious that the new policy has not made local coffee shops less attractive for tourists. Specially during the summer evenings, travelers under the influence of drugs are a frequent sight in any corner of De Wallen, Centrum, Jordaan, De Pijp, or the welcoming grass of the Vondelpark.

The visual aspect of their presence confirms indeed the sense of tolerance that surrounds the use of soft drugs in The Netherlands. But even if visitors do not sense it. Locals do experience nuisance and concerns rise among Dutchmen, according to media outlets, about what some have labeled a *narcostaat* (narco-state). Advertisement of either cannabis or coffee shops is not allowed, but the topic of soft drugs in the country permeates the visual realm in many other formats. From health campaign posters in schools to websites providing instructions on how to manipulate electricity cables in order to grow cannabis plants at home—without being billed additionally by the energy provider or caught by the police—*wiet* and *hasj* are part of the Dutch optical-social landscape. An example from television is the NTR-produced four-episode documentary *Narcostaat*, premiered in November 2019 and described by the producers as follows:

> *Narcostaat*: Tens of billions are lost in the drug industry, people are killed, officials are bribed, drug waste is dumped and more and more users are eagerly taking it. Who are the people behind the headlines and news stories? They are featured in this series. People from the above and from the underworld. Anonymous criminals—who normally seek out the shadows—now talk freely. Danny Ghosen talks to the cops who hunt them or experts who know a lot about the illegal world. And he talks to victims of the growing drug violence. (NTR, 2020)[21]

Screening the complex networks in which psychoactive substances are mobilized as commodities emphasizes the strength of human yearning to stimulate the mind. The ground for a quite profitable industry. A business that can weigh heavily on those affected by it. The brain and nervous system are the end stop and target destination of psychotropics, involving neurobiological and psychosocial factors that make the substance-body encounter simultaneously a health, social, and cultural matter. From a bioclusivity perspective, historical records confirm the use of mind-altering agents was (and is) part of the cultural practices and repertoire of many large civilizations and smaller nations. The tolerance policy of The Netherlands will be remembered as a pioneering approach to the dynamic between licit and illicit substances in a modern postindustrial society. While other countries have implemented similar or even more permissive legislations, the question remains to which degree *wiet* is part of Dutch culture or merely recreation or business.

To which extent is cannabis as a plant part of the bioclusivity order that underpins the relation between nature and health in The Netherlands? Or are the iconic green leaves displayed on coffee shops' paraphernalia only decoration? Soft drugs are drugs and have manifold reverberations. On the notion of *narcostaat*, Maris (2018) notes that although fighting serious crime should be a priority, "It must not burden consumers with guilt over the current messy state of affairs. Just out of respect for our national cultural heritage: the pragmatic Dutch tolerance" (68).[22] Maris's words prompt a reflection on whether regardless of the use or provenance (natural or artificial) of a practice or object, tolerance should prevail over any attempt to limit or restrict people's emancipation. A kind of freedom that resembles the immunity that lies behind the artistic creation of representations. An attitude that shows in images of cannabis plants in humorous designs on clothes, stickers, fridge magnets, postcards, and mugs sold, for instance, across Amsterdam as souvenirs and gifts. Another interpretation is that tolerance is part of Dutch mentality and should be applied to avoid any strategy to discipline the human mind. Even if economic interests, not a tradition of rebellion or tolerance, are probably the main reason, illegal networks based in The Netherlands do play a part in overruling efforts to prevent the use of narcotics. They do so by being some of the largest producers and traders of synthetic drugs (e.g., amphetamines) in the world. An approach illustratively encapsulated in hundreds of images of colorful *pilletjes* (pills) across the Internet, some displayed on the tip of the tongue of young people stuck out of their mouths.[23] The third interpretation of Maris's words relates to the notion of essence and, in specific, the capacity (and perhaps faculty) of Dutchmen to be open-minded. What might be considered an attitude grounded in the cultural memory and stored in the same minds that reject the idea of having restrictions on which substances they can have access to? It is then perhaps not a matter of cannabis or psychotropics in general, but about the free adoption and addition of objects and practices for those interested in interacting with them. If a nation's bioclusivity, as I argue, defines the relationship of its members with its habitat and the health ecosystems where they live, perhaps for the Dutchmen, freedom of choice is part of their (mental) medicinal repertoire or general well-being.

Another important aspect to consider is that mind-altering substances are a quite profitable source of income and that their prohibition has not dissipated the appetite of users and curiosity of potential consumers. If following the history of the propagation of stimulants (e.g., caffeine and nicotine), which serves as a predictor, the recent decriminalization of cannabis, mainly in the Americas, might signal a paradigm shift. It is possibly the onset of an era in which psychotropics become part of the biosocial repertoire of most countries. In nations, like Uruguay, where cannabis is legal since 2013, its visual presence across the Internet, print media, and public spaces grows progressively. Images of a notebook with the text "Si vas a estudiar, no consumas" (If you are going to study, don't consume) and a circular saw cutting wood tagged "Si vas a trabajar, no consumas" (If you are going to work, don't consume) are part of a project to promote a responsible consumption of the recreational substance.

In 2018, the Ministry of Public Health of Uruguay launched an awareness campaign, composed of four ad televised spots, with the motto "regular es ser responsible, dialogar sobre el tema también" (to regulate is to be responsible, and so is to talk about it). An initiative preceded by the #RESR campaign, launched by the National Drug Board and Institute for the Regulation and Control of Cannabis in 2017. While the 2018 campaign depicts scenes of daily life in which young people ask parents, teachers, and model figures about cannabis as a substance, the 2017 spots focus on legitimizing the decision behind the legalization. Publicly known and common Uruguayans explain briefly that "by regulating, we improve public health by reducing the damage associated with consumption." This final message is preceded by a voice-over that explains that regulating cannabis means saying "no to violence," "no to money laundering," "no to dealers," and "no to drug trafficking." The audiovisuals are brief but provide plenty of information about the health risks linked to consuming cannabis.[24] The psychotropic, as the spots make it clear, "alters perception, senses and reflexes," "in minors and pregnant women, its consumption is especially risky," and "limits the ability to concentrate and memory." Having average members of the community as spokespeople and tagging their daily occupation next to their first names gives the images a sense of intimacy and commitment. The four posters distributed throughout public places align with the main themes of the video: perils for pregnant women, work-related issues, the impact of cannabis on concentration, and the dangers of driving vehicles under the influence of the substance.

Cannabis is sold in the local pharmacies, and even though consumers complain that the official formulas are less potent than the ones sold in the black market, the legalization seems to be working.[25] As of September 2021, Uruguayan authorities are contemplating the option of allowing tourists to purchase cannabis locally. The question remains how effective the "open-door" policy (similar to the one adopted and discontinued in The Netherlands) will be. Alerting potential consumers about the risks involved in consuming cannabis for themselves and others is indexical of the health-related dimension of psychoactive precursors. Uruguay will probably provide consumers from overseas with enough information on the effect of cannabis on the human body. At the core of health communication lies its role of serving the community by informing them about the implications of practices and behaviors. A conscious addition (from a legal perspective) of cannabis, as in the case of Uruguay, and its social visibility suggest that biopsychosocial protocols are malleable, adaptable, and polymorphic. The legalization of the plant bears the earmarks of a historical moment in its process of de-stigmatization. A paradigm change that might introduce or modify how other societies perceive mind-altering compounds, eventually making adjustments to their canons and protocols. Plants endemic to geographies where local communities epistemologically understand disease, cure, religious beliefs, and spirituality in their own terms have been reformatted/reduced to isolated and often synthesized substances. Nonetheless, they have also become tangible, although morphologically diverse, evidence of how health and nature mutate as concepts, reflecting the impact of additions and transfers in the bioclusivity of the receptive community. Caring and curing for the body depend on the accumulation of health-related and medicinal knowledge, encompassing various agents and objects, transversed by multiple axes and spaces, the human mind being one of them, that once mobilized or activated, prompt new challenges.

NOTES

1. In the case of Ayahuasca tourism in Peru, some of the most images include psychedelic art, images of cooking pots, and photos of healers interacting with Western travelers.

2. Evidence shows use of psychoactive substances in prehistoric times, in various formats across the world, across genders, in combination with other substances, as commodities, as objects of self-experimentation and in lab contexts resulting eventually in applications in modern medicine (Lutsky et al., 1994; Berridge et al., 2007; Crocq, 2007; Tupper, 2008; Seddon, 2009; Kandall, 2010; Guerra-Doce, 2015; Hailwood, 2016; Winkelman and Winkelman, 2019).

3. For obvious reasons as the development of advanced drugs (Collins, 2011; Ayres et al., 2012; Carroll, 2012; O'Hagan and Smith, 2017; Evans-Brown and Sedefov, 2018; Tettey et al., 2018; Peacock et al., 2019), besides forcing new complex classifications (Zapata et al., 2021), is posing major concerns (Madras, 2016; Elliott et al., 2020) and creating illegal networks of circulation across the Internet (Jurásek, 2021).

4. Psychotropics production and distribution illicit networks in Colombia have lead the country to a civil war state, leaving massive ecological (Dávalos, 2018; Huezo, 2019; Rhodes at al., 2021) and sociopolitical marks (Andreas, 2019; Narvaez-Chicaiza). As is the case of Mexico, drug-related crimes have had tremendous consequences on the social fabric of both countries at all levels (Durán-Martínez, 2017). In Afghanistan, opium has impacted the livelihoods of millions, destabilizing fragile farming communities and fueling violence (Mansfield, 2016), whereas in Burma,

its cultivation has been linked to the militarization of the country in the form of counter-insurgency efforts (Lintner, 2019). The Netherlands was relatively successful in dealing with soft drug-related issues during the 1990s. Since the 2000s, matters concerning psychoactive substances are under jurisdiction of Security and Justice, instead of Heath authorities (Grund and Breeksema, 2017). A move that probably indicates the levels of criminality related to illicit hard drug circulation have considerably increased.

5. In fact, this second-wave psychedelic renaissance seems to be intensifying in depth and size (Sessa (2018); Kelly et al., 2019; George et al., 2020; Giffort, 2020; Holoyda, 2020; George et al., 2021: Hendy, 2021; Lu, 2021). Some advocate for a revolution that opens up spaces for underrepresented ethnic groups (George, 2020), while others warn about repeating mistakes from the past (Feinberg, 2018).

6. In 1928, German toxicologist Louis Lewin managed to isolate banisterine, today known as harmala alkaloid, the key main ingredient in ayahuasca. Finding the right name was problematic as he had desired to baptize it with a term that would allude to its telepathic properties. At some point, Lewin realized nevertheless that *Banisteriopsis caapi* derivatives did not endow their users with the power of reading minds. A valid observation again is the role of beliefs in inquisitive endeavors. At present, ayahuasca might be at the brink of becoming a therapeutic and pharmaceutical innovation (Sanabria, 2021), retaining its centrality and exceptionality at the heart of ayahuasca churches, mainly in Peru and Brazil, and ayahuasca tourism.

7. On psychotropics in Pre-Columbian Mesoamerica, Carod-Artal (2015) notes that "hallucinogenic cactus, plants and mushrooms were used to induce altered states of consciousness in healing rituals and religious ceremonies. The Maya drank balché (a mixture of honey and extracts of *Lonchocarpus*) in group ceremonies to achieve intoxication. Ritual enemas and other psychoactive substances were also used to induce states of trance. Olmec, Zapotec, Maya and Aztec used peyote, hallucinogenic mushrooms (teonanacatl: Psilocybe spp) and the seeds of ololiuhqui (*Turbina corymbosa*),that contain mescaline, psilocybin and lysergic acid amide, respectively. The skin of the toad Bufo spp contains bufotoxins with hallucinogenic properties, and was used since the Olmec period. Jimson weed (*Datura stramonium*), wild tobacco (Nicotiana rustica), water lily (*Nymphaea ampla*) and Salvia divinorum were used for their psychoactive effects. Mushroom stones dating from 3000 BC have been found in ritual contexts in Mesoamerica. Archaeological evidence of peyote use dates back to over 5000 years" (43).

8. Original text in Nahuatl and used as source for the translation: "pitzaoac, memecatic ixpitzaoac in jatlapalio: itoca ololiuhquj, teivinti, teiollomalacacho, teiolpolo, teiollotlavelilocatili, tetech qujneuh: in aqujn qujqua, in quj, mjec tlamantli qujtta in cenca temamauhti, vel mjhiçavia, coatl tequanj, tlein mach qujtta. In teococoliani: atl tlaqualli ipã qujtetololtia, injc teiollotlavelilotilia: iece xoiac, achi toxcacococ". Castilian Spanish version: "Hay una yerba que se llama coatlxoxouhqui, y cria una semilla que se dice ololiuhqui; esta semilla emborracha y enloquece, danla por bebedizos para hacer daño á los que quieren mal, y los que la comen paréceles que ven visiones y cosas espantables: danla á comer ó á beber, los hechiceros ó los que aborrecen á algunos para dáñarlos" (Porruca edition, 242).

9. In southern Mexico, López Ridaura (2015) observes that the plant is still used, as in pre-Columbian times, for curative and divinatory purposes (López Ridaura, 2015).

10. Dibble and Anderson, 1963, 129 (translation of *La Historia General de las Cosas de Nueva España/The Universal History of the Things* of *New Spain,* Book X1, Volume 7).

Original text: "PEIOTL: inin peiotl iztac: auh çan yio vmpa un mochioa intlacochcalcopa, in teutlapã in mjtoa mjetlanpa. In aqujnqujqua in, in anoço quj: itech qujça, iuhqujn nanacatl: no mjec tlamantli qujtta in temamauhti, anoço tevetzquijti aço cemjlhujtl, anoço omjlhujtl in jtech qujça, tel çan no concaoa: iece ca qujtlacoa in jiollo, tetlapololtia, teivintia, tetech qujça: njnopeiovia, njciovia." The text in Castilian Spanish reads: "Hay otra yerba como tunas de tierra, se llama peitol, es blanca, hácese ácia la parte del norte, los que la comen ó beben vén visiones espantosas ó irrisibles; dura esta borrachera dos ó tres dias y despues se quita; es comun manjar de los Chichimecas, pues los mantiene y da ánimo para pelear y no tender miedo, ni sed, ni hambre, y dicen que los guarda de todo peligro" (Sahagún, 1577, Book XI, Volume 7, p. 241 on the Porrua edition 1999).

11. Crown authorities stationed in the Americas implemented measurements against psychoactive agents also in Lima in 1629. For members of the inquisition, mind-altering substances were signals of "emploi diabolique" (diabolic work) (Boumediene, 2016, 340).

12. Once taking ingesting the buttons, Briggs (1887) alerts the scientific community about its effect on the heart: "Automatically I rushed to my able friend, Dr. E. J. Beall, of Fort Worth—my residence at the time. After giving him an idea, as best I could, of the trouble, he prescribed aro. spts. ammonia and whiskey, in large doses, every few minutes. This I took, if I remember right, one hour after having taken the "muscale button." It seemed necessary for me to walk in the open air for me to breathe. In about half an hour I felt some relief, and my pulse and respirations gradually became less until in about six or eight hours they were about normal. No bad consequences followed. I did, however, feel much depressed for about twelve hours—a feeling of malaise. The recollection of such experience is vividly impressed upon my mind. I believe if prompt aid had not been given me I should have died. . . . Whatever may be the ultimate constituents of this poison, it certainly is the most violent and rapid of all fruits, or even medicines, known to me—manifesting its first effects in less than fifteen minutes. I know of nothing like it except opium and cocaine. The most notable point is the rapidity with which it increases the heart's action. Next, the intoxication and subsequent depression. I think it well worth the trouble to investigate the matter. One man's experience is worth but little, and it is to be hoped some enterprising experimenter will carry out the research. As to myself, I must admit I feel somewhat abstemious on the subject" (145).

13. For instance, Bolivian torch cactus (*Echinopsis lageniformis*), San Pedro (*Echinopsis pachanoi*), and Peruvian torch (*Echinopsis peruviana/Trichocereus peruvianus*).

14. Jay (2019).

15. Advertisement of Peyote Tramni appeared in *La Démocratie*, *Le Journal*, *Le Matin*, *L'Œuvre* and *Le Tell* (one advertisement on June 24, 1933). In *Le Matin*, they

start appearing on a regular basis between February 16, 1932, and October, 1936, and in *L'Œuvre* for two years, between April 1935 and September 1937.

16. Other characteristics historically attributed to *maladie du scrupule* have included perfectionism, fear of self-confession and confusion between temptation and sin, often linked to sexual desire (Delumeau, 1983). Pierre Janet (1859–1947) did extensive work with patients presumably suffering from "scrupules" (scruple). He notes that shame and "mécontentement systématique" (systematic dissatisfaction) (1991, 357) are among the most salient symptoms. "Maladie du scrupule" or "des scrupules" is described to have paralyzing implications for those who suffer from it. From a young age, Thérèse of Lisieux (better known as Saint Therese of the Child Jesus and the Holy Face, 1873–1897) was one of those (self-diagnosed) patients believing to have this condition and be devastatingly affected by it. In her biography, Six (1998) observes that "C'est une véritable « maladie ». Le scrupuleux, dans son incapacité à arriver à la certitude morale, connaît la crainte, l'anxiété, tout particulièrement sur l'intégrité de ses confessions passées ; son état permanent d'angoisse et de culpabilité le traumatise gravement ; il n'arrive pas à porter un jugement objectif sur son agir ; il manifeste des comportements pathologiques : des récitations méticul" (It's a real "disease." The scrupulous, in his inability to arrive at moral certainty, knows fear, anxiety, especially on the integrity of his past confessions; his permanent state of anguish and guilt seriously traumatizes him; he is unable to pass an objective judgment on his to act; he manifests pathological behaviors: meticulous recitations) (16).

17. See Sabina and Pike (1957).

18. Sessa (2012).

19. This is an official translation, provided by the government, from the Dutch version that reads "Gedoogbeleid softdrugs en coffeeshops: Omdat softdrugs minder schadelijk zijn voor de gezondheid dan harddrugs, gelden hiervoor soms andere regels. Coffeeshops kunnen onder strenge voorwaarden wiet en hasj verkopen. Zij worden daarvoor niet strafrechtelijk vervolgd. Dit is de essentie van het gedoogbeleid. Ook vervolgt het Openbaar Ministerie personen niet als zij kleine hoeveelheden softdrugs bezitten" (Rijksoverhaid, 2021). Translation: "Tolerance policy for soft drugs and coffee shops: Because soft drugs are less harmful to health than hard drugs, different rules sometimes apply. Coffee shops can sell weed and hash under strict conditions. They will not be prosecuted for this. This is the essence of the tolerance policy. The Public Prosecution Service also does not prosecute people if they possess small amounts of soft drugs."

20. Rijksoverheid (2021).

21. Original text in Dutch: "In de drugsindustrie gaan tientallen miljarden om, er vallen doden, ambtenaren worden omgekocht, drugsafval wordt gedumpt én er wordt gretig afgenomen door steeds meer gebruikers. Wie zijn de mensen achter de krantenkoppen en nieuwsberichten? In deze serie komen ze aan het woord. Mensen uit de boven- én uit de onderwereld. Anonieme criminelen—die normaal de schaduw opzoeken—praten nu vrijuit. Danny Ghosen spreekt de agenten die op hen jagen of experts die veel weten van de illegale wereld. En hij praat met slachtoffers van het groeiende drugsgeweld" (NTR, 2020).

22. Full quote in its original version in Dutch: "Op de lange duur moet ze dat ook nastreven voor zwaardere drugs. Daarnaast blijft bestrijding van zware misdaad natuurlijk een centrale overheidstaak. Maar in de tussentijd moet ze consumenten niet opzadelen met schuldgevoel over de huidige rommelige stand van zaken. Alleen al uit eerbied voor ons nationale culturele erfgoed: de pragmatische Hollandse tolerantie" (Maris, 2018: 68). English translation: "In the long run, she should also strive for that for heavier drugs. In addition, combating serious crime naturally remains a central government task. But in the meantime, it must not burden consumers with guilt over the current messy state of affairs. Just out of respect for our national cultural heritage: the pragmatic Dutch tolerance" (Maris, 2018: 68).

23. These images are sometimes informally used as reference to public events (e.g., festivals).

24. Effect of cannabis on the body involves more organs and systems than the brain and nervous system, both positively and negatively (Ashton, 200; Iversen, 2005; Hall, 2019; Datta et al., 2021).

25. Laqueur et al. (2020) bases their conclusions on the consumption among adolescents before and after legalization.

Conclusion

The journey through images, decades (centuries in some cases), geographies, cosmologies, worldviews, customs, and beliefs has led me to confirm the importance of understanding how societies express and articulate semiotically the relation between health and the natural world. I have drawn on various formats of visual culture to review study cases from different parts of the globe. Throughout this book, the main argument has been that visual culture offers insights into how societies conceptualize the role of nature in their, and others', pursuit to cure and care for the human body. And that this happens in unique ways every time because the bios-society dynamic is equally unique in every case.

All along, scientific research, mostly through references to publications in medicine and pharmacology, has served to contextualize the framework of paradigms, which provides a description of the world I presume to understand: modern science. A body of knowledge, produced in every corner of the world, as the referenced papers in this book confirm, and in principle, united by comparable and, ideally, rigorous epistemic practices. Evidence-based findings, fruits of meticulous application of scientific methodologies and instruments, reproductible, universal, and discardable only in light of new evidence, do not, however, I posit, offer the *full picture*—pun intended—of how cultures imagine the connection between nature and health. I suggest that each community develops its own sense of what I call bioclusivity: an intimate mindset and understanding of the natural world, accessible through externalizations and representations to outsiders, but only truly decipherable and coherent to those immersed in it. "Clusivity" is a term borrowed from linguistics. It refers to the faculty of language to distinguish between, for instance, inclusive we and exclusive we. "We (she and I) go to the party" is different in meaning from "we (you and I) go to the party." The connotation of both sentences and the distinction between them is a product of the embedded or previous knowledge of the interlocutor. To the uninformed mind, both sentences might look or sound the same. Some languages mark clusivity through pronouns and verb declensions, but in all cases, it is, of course, compelling to know the language in order to comprehend what is being said. In similar ways, I claim that each community has developed its own set of codes to relate to its surroundings, by default, including and excluding those who are or are not proficient in it. Bioclusivity is the particular blueprint through which a society has imprinted nature in its own *cultural DNA*. This imprinting process has integrated the notion of health for obvious reasons. Humans, regardless of their ontological definition of life, have an instinct for survival and that involves surviving illness.

From time immemorial, the presence of disease and injury has left marks in human culture, much of it documented through material objects, inherited practices, historical records, oral history and visual representations. Works of art as expressions of emotions, values, reactions, and sensitivities have registered the dominant views about health and nature at the time of their creation. Some examples reviewed in the introduction illustrate the nexus between medicine, nature, and culture in epistemic-semiotic renderings enacted through formats that range from petroglyphs to modern-day consumables packaging. Unknown illustrators, as well as highly celebrated known artists, have found inspiration in the nature-health dyad, and by extension, as I claim, in their own bioclusivity.

On this account, visual representations can be appreciated for their reportorial qualities, but also as objects with their own historical value. Yet, creation, circulation, and preservation of visual renderings, reflections, and critiques, in particular, before the introduction of tools, such as photography, have not been within reach of large segments of the human population. More importantly, visual and material cultures have operated differently across the globe. Assuming that art exists as a fixed concept or operationalization of human expression universally is a sign of short-sightedness. The survival of objects or their conservation does not guarantee the availability of enough tools to understand the evolution and circulation of ideas across time and space. The importance of history lies in its capacity of reenacting modes of reencountering our own past, disclosing, and unraveling the mysteries, paradoxes, and lines of events that have anticipated and reshaped present-day attitudes, practices, and state of affairs. Health and nature, as concepts, have shifted meaning in light of social, economic, political, and as it is happening at the moment, environmental upheavals, crises, and revolutions. All along, knowledge production has defined much of the development of medicine, first as an art (many still consider it an artform), eventually as practical operationalization of scientific discoveries. Targeted experimentation, extensive collaborations, celebrated accidents, random guesses, and unrelentless pursuit for a better understanding of natural phenomena have paved the road for the institutionalization of modern science. Much about the human body remains a secret, but twenty-first-century biomedicine advances in a steadier and more efficient way than ever before in history. Knowledge about the body has served as content and context for epistemic transfers across cultures and geographies, often engendered in tangible artifacts and intangible practices. Circulation of ideas and mobilization of objects have reshaped epistemic systems and regimes. Objects have included not only manmade devices but also commodities, such as medicinal plants of all sorts. Both the circulation and encounters have left traces in the knowledge system of their transporters and the visual culture of their recipients.

The introduction of technological advances ignites reconfigurations that progressively become solidified parts of the legacy and heritage of a community. In terms of health-oriented innovations, drastic changes in the biosocial landscape have at various points accelerated the adoption of new tools, protocols, and paradigms. Health concerns touch upon most other aspects of social life. Even if there is perhaps no consensus on its definition, there is a consensus of its ubiquity throughout every human's lifetime. The inclusion of health as a theme and genre in visual culture has partly to do with the urgency of disseminating or promoting knowledge about medical issues. In the twenty-first century, medicine-related axioms account for a significant portion of science communication outputs, platforms, and outreach channels. The progressive growth and development of formats to mediate knowledge about health have grown exponentially. Visual and textual references about prevention, diagnosis, and treatment of pathologies, illnesses, conditions, viruses, infections, and affections abound in contemporary media outlets. This does not mean they all inform and communicate. A portion of it misinforms and miscommunicates. There has never been more social participation in the creation and maintenance of mass media outputs as is the case today. On the one hand, this has allowed for the expansion of uncorroborated information and alternative facts. Examples of these include the infographics discussed in chapter 3.

On the other hand, the contemporary landscape of images presumably provides good insights into the series of attitudes and assumptions societies hold about the cure and care of the body and the natural world. As I show, nature and health, and the interface of the two, are visual topics found in fiction films and documentaries (chapter 1); over-the-counter health-enhancing consumables, remedies, supplements, and nutraceuticals (chapter 3); natural cosmeceuticals (chapter 4); public spaces (chapter 5); and more specialized locations (chapter 6). As chapter 2 shows, they are also themes identified in toys, animated series, and books. Due to the targeted audiences, they confirm the role of media in processes of cultural leveling, education, socialization, and maintenance of epistemic systems and ontological regimes. What all the chapters have in common is an urge to shed light on the visual-material dimension of objects and cultural artifacts that do not routinely inform academic discussions about science, naturality (the state of being natural), and health. I hope this book has managed to show that an old movie, a moringa milkshake, a lipstick, a children's book, a post on social media, a short-length vlog, a day by the pool, and a *joint* play a role in the visual construction of ideas about health and the natural world. These objects seem trivial and transient, and yet, as the stories behind them show, they hold an epistemic value and engender cultural practices that register how their producers and users imagine the role of nature as a panacea. Trivial objects matter precisely because they are part of the daily routines of millions around the globe. In an ailing planet, on the brink of an ecological catastrophe, it is crucial to understand how different our relations are toward nature and the spaces we inhabit. While the first image of a black hole in space makes history for many well-deserved reasons, places much closer to us, such as the kitchen and bathroom, might deserve to be part of the history of science as well.

The knowledge behind the production of consumables and everyday objects retains its epistemic value even if those objects become commonplace. The context in which raw materials and finite products navigate oceans is equally worth exploring to understand what societies value. Understanding the commercialization of health as an industry and of nature as an infinite fountain of resources involves scrutinizing, for instance, the trivialization of a plant farmed in Madagascar that serves to create the illusion of beauty in a South Korean lab and a German cosmetic store. A superfood from Peru for breakfast in Russia is equally a matter worth exploring in more detail in order to understand how the tripartite health-nature-culture defines modern lives. Health is not a trivial matter and yet, much of what encompasses the construction of healthier lifestyles comes from relatively small practices and apparently insignificant choices.

If our own bioclusivity, as I see it, informs our ontological awareness and knowingness about our environments, it seems obvious to me that we need to be proficient in more than one bioclusivity system, if the goal is to save the Earth. The *healthy* thing to do is to comprehend what nature means for others and how others assume it contributes to their own survival (the ultimate goal of caring for our bodies). Behaviors, customs, and ideas are cornerstones of culture. Out of the three, the notion of ideas plays a special role in the construction of affiliation and cohesion within societies. Few outlets exemplify this situation better than the creation of visual externalizations of one's modus vivendi, habitat, or utopias. Depicting health and nature involves choosing which elements matter and which ones can be discarded. Portrayals of health, as many of the images discussed in this book show, require taking a stand about what it means to be free of disease and injury. There seems to be a tendency to idealize nature as a precursor to the restoration and maintenance of healthy bodies and minds. Utopic scenarios, like those sketched in fiction, animation, and overinflated infographics, discussed in chapters 1 and 2, and on labels of health-enhancing natural supplements and skincare products, explored in chapters 3 and 4, confirm we are ready to believe nature holds all answers. Commonalities about certain aspects do not mean the underlying forces that underpin the bios-*Homo sapiens* interconnection does not differ considerably about other aspects across the planet.

Avoiding essentialist readings of their culture, there is a stark contrast between Indigenous and non-Indigenous, industrialized societies. It seems to be a matter of observing different ontological and epistemological frameworks, and perhaps also a question of urban versus rural lifestyles, spiritual and religious values, or having a history of colonization. Videos produced by Indigenous communities or made in collaboration with them as informants, according to my findings, imbue perceptual awareness of the body as an extension of the places where the corporal lives and thrives. In fact, humans cannot expect to live and thrive unless they create conditions that do not cause disarray in the ecosystems where they have settled. While some Indigenous communities use media outlets to share their cosmovision, there are aspects they consider to be the domain only of those who belong to the community. Medicinal practices take place in the context of direct interaction between healers and patients (not clients) and, simultaneously, of synergic instances between the medicine people and a spiritual world only perceptible to them. By means of the narratives Indigenous medicine people agree to share, it is noticeable that the existence of the intangible and invisible signal and inform their cosmovision in general terms, and in particular, in their daily activities as health agents of their communities.

Some differences are observable in their approach to plants as ingredients for preparations and plants as tokens of consecration and belief. The social hierarchy, observed by most countries, that situates biomedicine above any other medicinal praxis or biosocial epistemic system is a well-known fact to the practitioners of Indigenous medicine. For the couple of Okanagan medicine people discussed in chapter 5, each medicine has a place and a time. For Kaqchikel *ajq'ij* (spiritual guide), knowledge of Mayan ancient traditions is impendent to create healing and preventive protocols for their patients. An interesting aspect of the cinematic/mediatic presence of Indigenous medicine people is their eagerness to share their knowledge with any potential viewer. From this perspective, the recorded videos become archival material and documented sources of the teachings these healers consider worth diffusing among members from outside their communities. This choice can be seen from many viewpoints.

First, visual culture outlets might offer the visibility that the above-mentioned hierarchical structures hamper in terms of outreach. Second, medicine people working outside monetized systems in which human health is an industry, see dissemination of knowledge as a contribution to everyone's well-being, as opposed to a service. In fact, in the Okanagan tradition, charging is not allowed. The only retributions are offerings in the form of, for instance, tobacco or sweetgrass. Third, their willingness to discuss openly in which ways their medicinal practices bear little resemblance with biomedicine denotes their awareness of the differences between Indigenous and non-Indigenous medicine. They do not speak of one system in opposition to the other at any moment. Quite the opposite, some Indigenous medicine practitioners regret that biomedicine professionals do not show interest in collaborating with them. Methodologically, both Okanagan and Mayan medical traditions, as they are presented in the reviewed films, involve practices that cannot always be supported by scientific evidence. In terms of diagnosis and treatment, any emphasis on spirituality and allusions to a superior being/force are diametrically inverse to the grounding basis of modern Western medicine. Para-, proto-, pre-, and pseudo-scientific labels denote in themselves considerable differences in the definition of what health is, when disease is absent, and how to treat and prevent it.

Nature as an idea is found in artifacts that visually reflect the interplay between the realms of imagination, health, and culture, as much as the commodification and capitalization of resources, political power, and inequality at a global scale. Living organisms, such as plants and animals, are morphologically conditioned to formats that can be adapted to the logistics and economics of consuming societies. A bowl of spirulina powder seems trivial, but when it is sold in a Finnish supermarket, manufactured in The Netherlands, with algae from Chad, and marketed by creating links between the potentiality of *dihe*, as is known locally in Chad, to restore and enhance human health, it ceases to be *just* an algae.

In the large context, I posit that charting how communities and individuals understand, imagine, envision, perceive, and regard health and nature matters to tackle many of the challenges that we face in current times. In a world simultaneously overpowered by an ongoing ecological and sanitary crisis, it is crucial to reach a consensus on how to care for the planet and for the citizens that inhabit it. Since externalizations of assumptions and attitudes, and above all, imaginaries and ideas, register insiders' perspectives, they offer unvaluable data about their creators and potential audiences. Presumably, those aspects of the rapport between communities, their ecosystems, and health practices materialize in epistemic semiotic formats *because* they matter to the societies involved. Knowledge about medicinal practices, as mundane and questionable as they might seem, is as important as any other body of knowledge. As I hope this book has shown, time has come to understand that ontological differences are not criteria for the creation of epistemic hierarchies but a starting point of epistemological dialogues that recognize everyone's epistemic presence.

References

Aamyinaarrone aabhidharan / အမြင်အာရုံအဘိဓာန်. 2018. Yangon.

Abad Iglesias, Rafael. 1991. *US Patent WO1992015276A3: Therapeutic and Cosmetic Compositions for Treatment of Skin.* Washington, DC: U.S. Patent and Trademark Office.

Academia de Lenguas Mayas de Guatemala (ALMG). 2015.

Adams, Vincanne. 2001. "The Sacred in the Scientific: Ambiguous Practices of Science in Tibetan Medicine." *Cultural Anthropology* 16 (4): 542–575.

Adamson, Peter. 2019. "Introduction." In *Health: A History,* edited by Peter Adamson, 1–6. Oxford: Oxford University Press.

Adom, Muhammad Bahrain, Muhammad Taher, Muhammad Fathiy Mutalabisin, Mohamad Shahreen Amri, Muhammad Badri Abdul Kudos, Mohd Wan Azizi Wan Sulaiman, Pinaki Sengupta, and Deny Susanti. 2017. "Chemical Constituents and Medical Benefits of Plantago Major." *Biomedicine & Pharmacotherapy* 96: 348–360.

Agich, George. 1983. "Disease and Value: A Rejection of the Value-Neutrality Thesis." *Theoretical Medicine* 4: 27–41.

Ahuja, Akash, Ji Hye Kim, Jong-Hoon Kim, Young-Su Yi, and Jae Youl Cho. 2018. "Functional Role of Ginseng-derived Compounds in Cancer." *Journal of Ginseng Research* 42 (3): 248–254.

Ahuja, Kunal, and Sonal Singh. 2018. *Ginseng Extract Market.* Selbyville, DE: Global Market Insights.

Ajmone-Marsan, Paolo, Jose Fernando Garcia, and Johannes A. Lenstra. 2010. "On the Origin of Cattle: How Aurochs became Cattle and Colonized the World." *Evolutionary Anthropology: Issues, News, and Reviews* 19 (4): 148–157.

Alam, Eman. 2011. "Evaluation of Antioxidant and Antibacterial Activities of Egyptian *Maydis Stigma* (*Zea Mays* Hairs) Rich in Some Bioactive Constituents." *Journal of American Science* 7 (4): 726–729.

Alexandratos, Jonathan. 2017. *Articulating the Action Figure.* Jefferson, NC: McFarland.

Alfonse, Marco, and Mariam Gawich. 2020. "Ontologies on Biomedical Informatics." In *Ontology-Based Information Retrieval for Healthcare Systems*, edited by Vishal Jain, Ritika Wason, Jyotir Moy Chatterjee, and Dac-Nhuong Le, 233–244. New York, NY: Wiley.

Al-Haddad, Shafig, Alaa Awad, Diala Albate, Ibrahim Almashhadani, and Wasan Dirani. 2020. "Factors Affecting Green Cosmetics Purchase Intention." *Journal of Management Information and Decision Sciences* 23 (4): 332–342.

Alsayari, Abdulrhman, Abdullatif Bin Muhsinah, Dalia Almaghaslah, Sivakumar Annadurai, and Shadma Wahab. 2021. "Pharmacological Efficacy of Ginseng against Respiratory Tract Infections." *Molecules* 26 (13): 4095.

Alubala, Agneta. 2018. "Effects of Facebook Advertising on Cosmetics Sales and Purchase by Women in Kenya." Diss. University of Nairobi.

Alþingi. 1940. *Frumvarp til íþróttalaga.*

Anati, Emanuel. 2001. *Gobustan: Azerbaijan.* Capo di Ponte: Edizione del Centro.

Anderson, Eugene. 2010. "Food Cultures: Linking People to Landscapes." In *Nature and Culture*, edited by Sarah Pilgrim and Jules Pretty, 185–196. London: Earthscan.

Andreas, Peter. 2019. "Drugs and War: What Is the Relationship?" *Annual Review of Political Science* 22: 57–73.

Andresen, Georg Julius. 1875. *Die Wasserkur in ihrer Stellung zur Heilkraft des Organismus und zur ärztlichen Kunst.* Berlin: Verlag von August Hirschwald.

Antioco, Michael, Dirk Smeesters, and Aline Le Boedec. 2012. "Take Your Pick: Kate Moss or the Girl Next Door?: The Effectiveness of Cosmetics Advertising." *Journal of Advertising Research* 52 (1): 15–30.

Appiah, Kwame Anthony. 2018. *The Lies that Bind: Rethinking Identity.* London: Profile Books.

Apud Peláez, Ismael Eduardo. 2020. *Ayahuasca: Between Cognition and Culture: Perspectives from an Interdisciplinary and Reflexive Ethnography.* Tarragona: Publicaciones URV.

Archer, Patricia. 1989. "From the Beginning: An Historical Review of Medical Art." *Journal of Audiovisual Media in Medicine* 12 (2): 51–62.

Artz, Lee. 2015. "Animating Transnational Capitalism." *Journal of Intercultural Communication Research* 44 (2): 93–107.

Ashton, C. Heather. 2001. "Pharmacology and Effects of Cannabis: A Brief Review." *The British Journal of Psychiatry* 178 (2): 101–106.

Asquith, Kyle. 2021. "The Visual Clichés of Legal Cannabis Promotion on Social Media." *Critical Studies in Media Communication* 38 (4): 336–349.

Augstein, Hannah Franziska. 1999. *James Cowles Prichard's Anthropology: Remaking the Science of Man in Early Nineteenth-century Britain.* Vol. 52. Amsterdam: Rodopi.

Ayres, Tammy C., and John W. Bond. 2012. "A Chemical Analysis Examining the Pharmacology of Novel Psychoactive Substances Freely Available over the Internet and their Impact on Public (Ill) Health. Legal Highs or Illegal Highs?." *BMJ Open* 2 (4): e000977.

Baggio, Guilherme, Manzoor Qadir, and Vladimir Smakhtin. 2021. "Freshwater Availability Status Across Countries for Human and Ecosystem Needs." *Science of the Total Environment* 792: 148230.

Bahadoran, Parvin. 2009. "Exploring the role of Midwives in Health Care System in Iran and the World." *Iranian Journal of Nursing and Midwifery Research* 14 (3): 117–122.

Bai, Zhihong. 2018. "The Characteristics of Language in Cosmetic Advertisements." *Theory and Practice in Language Studies* 8 (7): 841–847.

Banerjee, Debanjan, and Kolar Meena. 2021. "COVID-19 as an 'Infodemic' in Public Health: Critical Role of the Social Media." *Frontiers in Public Health* 9: 231.

Banerjee, Madhulika. 2002. "Power, Culture and Medicine: Ayurvedic Pharmaceuticals in the Modern Market." *Contributions to Indian Sociology* 36 (3): 435–467.

Bánki, Judit, ed. 2010. *Képes Magyar értelmező szótár*. Budapest: Akadémiai Kiadó.

Bard, Jonathan. 2003. "Ontologies: Formalising Biological Knowledge for Bioinformatics." *Bioessays* 25 (5): 501–506.

Barkemeyer, Ralf, Philippe Givry, and Frank Figge. 2018. "Trends and Patterns in Sustainability-related Media Coverage: A Classification of Issue-level Attention." *Environment and Planning C: Politics and Spac*e 36 (5): 937–962.

Barnes, Bradley, and Maki Yamamoto. 2008. "Exploring International Cosmetics Advertising in Japan." *Journal of Marketing Management* 24 (3–4): 299–316.

Barnes, Bradley R., Philip J. Kitchen, Graham Spickett-Jones, and Qionglei Yu. 2004. "Investigating the Impact of International Cosmetics Advertising in China." *International Journal of Advertising* 23 (3): 361–387.

Batkin, Jane. 2017. *Identity in Animation: A Journey into Self. Difference, Culture and the Body*. New York: Routledge.

Baumans, Vera. 2004. "Use of Animals in Experimental Research: An Ethical Dilemma?." *Gene Therapy* 11 (1): S64–S66.

Baumgarten, Alfred. 2015 (1898). *Sebastian Kneipp. Biografie*. Hamburg: Severus.

Beinart, William, and Karen Brown. 2013. *African Local Knowledge & Livestock Health: Diseases & Treatments in South Africa*. Woodbridge: Boydell & Brewer.

Bekiari, Maria, Paris Iakovidis, Dimitrios Lytras, Ioanna P. Chatziprodromidou, and Eleftherios Dimitros. 2021. "The Effect of Hydrotherapy on the Symptoms and Functional Characteristics of Multiple Sclerosis Patients." *International Journal of Physical Education, Sports and Health* 8 (2): 191–197.

Benbow-Buitenhuis, Anoushka. 2014. "A Feminine Double-bind?: Towards Understanding the Commercialisation of Beauty through Examining Anti-Ageing Culture." *Social Alternatives* 33 (2): 43–49.

Benoit, Cecilia, Sirpa Wrede, Ivy Bourgeault, Jane Sandall, Raymond De Vries, and Edwin van Teijlingen. 2005. "Understanding the Social Organisation of Maternity Care Systems: Midwifery as a Touchstone." *Sociology of Health and Illness* 27 (6): 722–737.

Bent, Stephen. 2008. "Herbal Medicine in the United States: Review of Efficacy, Safety, and Regulation." *Journal of General Internal Medicine* 23 (6): 854–859.

Bergmann, Gunnar. 1964. "Á endaspretti með Þórberqi." *Tíminn*, March 12, 1964.

Berridge, Virginia, and Tim Hickman. 2007. "History and the Future of Psychoactive Substances." In *Drugs and the Future*, edited by David Nutt, Trevor W. Robbins, Gerald V. Stimson, Martin Ince, and Andrew Jackson, 467–483. London: Academic Press.

Berry, Nicole. 2006. "Kaqchikel Midwives, Home Births, and Emergency Obstetric Referrals in Guatemala: Contextualizing the Choice to Stay at Home." *Social Science & Medicine* 62 (8): 1958–1969.

Berryman, Rachel, and Misha Kavka. 2017. "'I Guess a Lot of People See Me as a Big Sister or a Friend': The Role of Intimacy in the Celebrification of Beauty Vloggers." *Journal of Gender Studies* 26 (3): 307–320.

Biagioli, Mario. 1990. "The Anthropology of Incommensurability." *Studies in History and Philosophy of Science* 21 (2): 183–209.

Bian, He. 2014. "Assembling the Cure: Materia Medica and the Culture of Healing in Late Imperial China." PhD diss., Harvard University.

Biermayr-Jenzano, Patricia, Shinan N. Kassam, and Aden Aw-Hassan. 2014. "Understanding Gender and Poverty Dimensions of High Value Agricultural Commodity Chains in the Souss-Masaa-Draa Region of Southwestern Morocco." ICARDA Working Paper. Amman, Jordan.

Birla, Nikhlesh, and Sumeet Dwivedi. 2020. "*Stigma Maydis*: A Promising Traditional Therapeutic Herb." *Journal of Advanced Scientific Research* 11: 16–24.

Bishop, William John, and Norman Murdoch Matheson. 1948. *Medicine and Science in Postage Stamps*. London: Harvey & Blythe.

Biswas, Dew, Samapika Nandy, Anuradha Mukherjee, Devendra Kumar Pandey, and Abhijit Dey. 2020. "Moringa Oleifera Lam. and Derived Phytochemicals as Promising Antiviral Agents: A Review." *South African Journal of Botany* 129: 272–282.

Bivins, Roberta. 2007. *Alternative Medicine?* London: A History. Oxford University.

Bjarnason, Egill. 29 October 2017. "Sundlaugistan." *Morgunblaðið.*

Björkqvist, Kaj, and Kristi Lagerspetz. 1985. "Children's Experience of Three Types of Cartoons at Two Age Levels." *International Journal of Psychology* 20: 77–93.

Black, Rebecca, Bill Tomlinson, and Ksneia Korobkova. 2016. "Play and Identity in Gendered LEGO® Franchises." *International Journal of Play* 5 (1): 64–76.

Blanco-Dávila, Feliciano. 2000. "Beauty and the Body: The Origins of Cosmetics." *Plastic and Reconstructive Surgery* 105 (3): 1196–1204.

Bleichmar, Daniela, and Vanessa R. Schwartz. 2019. "Visual History: The Past in Pictures." *Representations* 145 (1): 1–31.

Blome, Christine, Marc A. Radtke, Leah Eissing, and Matthias Augustin. 2016. "Quality of Life in Patients with Atopic Dermatitis: Disease Burden, Measurement, and Treatment Benefit." *American Journal of Clinical Dermatology* 17 (2): 163–169.

Bonah, Christian, and Anja Laukötter. 2020. "Introduction." In *Body, Capital, and Screens: Visual Media and the Healthy Self in the 20th Century,* 13–38. Amsterdam: Amsterdam University Press.

Bonell, Sarah, Fiona Kate Barlow, and Scott Griffiths. 2021. "The Cosmetic Surgery Paradox: Toward a Contemporary Understanding of Cosmetic Surgery Popularisation and Attitudes." *Body Image* 38: 230–240.

Bonnemain, Bruno. 2005. "Helix and Drugs: Snails for Western Health Care from Antiquity to the Present." *Evidence-Based Complementary and Alternative Medicine* 2 (1): 25–28.

Boumediene, Samir. 2016. *La colonisation du savoir: Une histoire des plantes médicinales du « Nouveau Monde » (1492–1750).* Vaulx-en-Velin: Éditions des Mondes à faire.

Bradford, Clare. 2007. *Unsettling Narratives: Postcolonial Readings of Children's Literature.* Waterloo: Wilfrid Laurier University Press.

Brandt, Fredric S., Alex Cazzaniga, and Michael Hann. 2011. "Cosmeceuticals: Current Trends and Market Analysis." *Seminars in Cutaneous Medicine and Surgery* 3: 141–143.

Briggs, John Raleigh. 1887. "Muscale Buttons' Physiological Effects Personal Experience." *The Medical Bulletin*: 144–145.

Brown, Kerri. 2016. "The Use of Medicinal Plants in Rio de Janeiro's Urban Periphery: An Analysis of Communities' Engagements with Policies." *Societies of Ethnobiology* 36 (4): 861–880.

Brumm, Adam, Adhi Agus Oktaviana, Basran Burhan, Budianto Hakim, Rustan Lebe, Jian-Xin Zhao, Priyatno Hadi Sulistyarto, Marlon Ririmasse, Shinatria Adhityatama, Iwan Sumantri, and Maxime Aubert. 2021. "Oldest Cave Art Found in Sulawesi." *Science Advances* 7 (3): eabd4648. doi: 10.1126/sciadv.abd4648.

Buchanan, Scott. 1938. *The Doctrine of Signatures.* London: Routledge.

Cairo, Alberto. 2012. *The Functional Art: An Introduction to Information Graphics and Visualization.* London: Harrow.

Cairo, Alberto. 2020. "Foreword: The Dawn of a Philosophy of Visualization." In *Data Visualization in Society*, 17–18. Amsterdam: Amsterdam University Press.

Çakmur, Hülya, and Emine Derviş. 2015. "The Relationship between Quality of Life and the Severity of Psoriasis in Turkey." *European Journal of Dermatology* 25 (2): 169–176.

Calkins, Casey M., James P. Franciosi, and Gary L. Kolesari. 1999. "Human Anatomical Science and Illustration: The Origin of Two Inseparable Disciplines." *Clinical Anatomy* 12 (2): 120–129.

Campo, Laurentino Lucas. 2018. "Conocimientos de los makuchinanin Tutunakú en Huehuetla, Puebla, México." *Etnobiología* 16 (2): 5–17.

Carod-Artal, Francisco Javier. 2015. "Hallucinogenic Drugs in Pre-Columbian Mesoamerican Cultures." *Neurología* 30 (1): 42–49.

Carroll, Ivy, Anita Lewin, Wayne Mascarella, Herbert H. Seltzman, and Anantha Reddy. 2012. "Designer Drugs: A Medicinal Chemistry Perspective." *Annals of the New York Academy of Sciences* 1248 (1): 18–38.

Cawte, John. 1985. "Psychoactive Substances of the South Seas: Betel, Kava and Pituri." *Australian and New Zealand Journal of Psychiatry* 19 (1): 83–87.

Charmaz, Kathy. 1991. *Good Days, Bad Days: The Self in Chronic Illness and Time.* New Brusnwick, NJ: Rutgers University Press.

Charrouf, Zoubida, and Guillaume Don. 1999. "Ethnoeconomical, Ethnomedical and Phytochemical Study of *Argania spinosa* (L.) Skeels." *Journal of Ethnopharmacology* 67: 7–14.

Charrouf, Zoubida, and Guillaume Don. 2011. "Argan Oil and Other Argan Products: Use in Dermocosmetology." *European Journal of Lipid Science and Technology* 11 (113): 403–408.

Chary, Anita, Anne Kraemer Díaz, Brent Henderson, and Peter Rohloff. 2013. "The Changing Role of Indigenous Lay Midwives in Guatemala: New Frameworks for Analysis." *Midwifery* 29 (8): 852–858.

Chen, Min-Hung, Kai-Min Yang, Tzou-Chi Huang, and Mei-Li Wu. 2017. "Traditional Small-size Citrus from Taiwan: Essential Oils, Bioactive Compounds and Antioxidant Capacity." *Medicines* 4 (2): 28.

Cherki, Mounia, Hicham Berrougui, Anas Drissi, Ahmed Adlouni, and Abdelouahed Khalil. 2006. "Argan Oil: Which Benefits on Cardiovascular Diseases?" *Pharmacological Research* 54 (1): 1–5.

Cho, Gayoung, Hyo-Min Park, Won-Mo Jung, Woong-Seok Cha, Donghun Lee, and Younbyoung Chae. 2020. "Identification of Candidate Medicinal Herbs for Skincare via Data Mining of the Classic Donguibogam Text on Korean Medicine." *Integrative Medicine Research* 9 (4): 10043.

Choi, Jae-Hwan, Hyoung-Man Kim, Young-Sook Song, Sun-Gyoo Park, Jin-Jun Kim, and Cheon-Koo Lee. 2007. "Anti-aging Effects Saccharomyces Fermented Modified Kyungohkgo Extract on Skin." *The Korea Journal of Herbology* 22 (4): 219–225.

Choi, JungBong, and Roald Maliangkay, eds. 2015. *K-pop: The International Rise of the Korean Music Industry*. Vol. 40. London: Routledge.

Christensen, Søren Brøgger. 2021. "Natural Products That Changed Society." *Biomedicines* 9 (5): 472.

Cilia, Giovanni, and Filippo Fratini. 2018. "Antimicrobial Properties of Terrestrial Snail and Slug Mucus." *Journal of Complementary and Integrative Medicine* 15 (3): 20170168.

Cimino, James J., and Xinxin Zhu. 2006. "The Practical Impact of Ontologies on Biomedical Informatics." *Yearbook of Medical Informatics* 15 (1): 124–135.

Clarke, David. 1963. "Effect of Immersion in Hot and Cold Water Upon Recovery of Muscular Strength following Fatiguing Isometric Exercise." *Archives of Physical Medicine and Rehabilitation* 44: 565–568.

Clarke, David, and George Stelmach. 1966. "Muscular Fatigue and Recovery Curve Parameters at Various Temperatures." *Research Quarterly. American Association for Health, Physical Education and Recreation* 37 (4): 468–479.

Clarke, Edward Daniel. 1848. *Travels in Russia, Tartary, and Turkey.* Aberdeen: Clark and Son.

Clarke, Jack, Jukka Heinonen, and Juudit Ottelin. 2017. "Emissions in a Decarbonised Economy? Global Lessons from a Carbon Footprint Analysis of Iceland." *Journal of Cleaner Production* 166: 1175–1186.

Clouser, Danner, Charles Culver, and Bernard Gert. 1981. "Malady: A New Treatment of Disease." *The Hastings Center* Report 11: 29–37.

Cockram, Sarah, and Andrew Wells. 2017. *Interspecies Interactions: Animals and Humans between the Middle Ages and Modernity.* London: Taylor & Francis.

Collins, Cecilia. 2020. "Tuberculosis in Medieval Iceland: Evidence from Hofstaðir, Keldudalur and Skeljastaðir." *Homo* 71 (4): 299–316.

Collins, Michael. 2011. "Some New Psychoactive Substances: Precursor Chemicals and Synthesis-driven End-products." *Drug Testing and Analysis* 3 (7–8): 404–416.

Congreso de Guatemala. 1997. *Codigo De Salud, Decreto Numero 90–97*. Ciudad de Guatemala: Congreso de la República de Guatemala.

Cooper, Rachel. 2005. *Classifying Madness*. Vol. 86. Dordrecht: Springer.

Cooper, Richard J. 2013. "Over-the-counter Medicine Abuse–A Review of the Literature." *Journal of Substance Use* 18 (2): 82–107.

Cornet, Ronald, and Ameen Abu-Hanna. 2003. "Using Description Logics for Managing Medical Terminologies." In *Conference on Artificial Intelligence in Medicine in Europe*, 61–70. Berlin: Springer.

Cosminsky, Sheila. 2021. *Midwives and Mothers: The Medicalization of Childbirth on a Guatemalan Plantation*. New York, NY: University of Texas Press.

Coughlin, Maura, and Emily Gephart, eds. 2020. *Ecocriticism and the Anthropocene in Nineteenth-century Art and Visual Culture*. London-New York: Routledge.

Counihan, Carole. 2009. *A Tortilla Is Like Life: Food and Culture in the San Luis Valley of Colorado*. Austin: University of Texas Press.

Cox, Robert. 2013. *Environmental Communication and the Public Sphere*. Los Angeles: Sage.

Craw, Charlotte. 2008. "The Flavours of the Indigenous: Branding Native Food Products in Contemporary Australia." *Sites* 5 (1): 41–62.

Craw, Charlotte. 2012. "Gustatory Redemption?" *International Journal of Critical Indigenous Studies* 5 (2): 13–24.

Crawford, Matthew James. 2016. *The Andean Wonder Drug: Cinchona Bark and Imperial Science in the Spanish Atlantic, 1630–1800*. Pittsburgh: University of Pittsburgh Press.

Crawford, Stephanie Y., and Catherine Leventis. 2005. "Herbal Product Claims: Boundaries of Marketing and Science." *Journal of Consumer Marketing* 22: 432–436.

Crocq, Marc-Antoine. 2007. "Historical and Cultural Aspects of Man's Relationship with Addictive Drugs." *Dialogues in Clinical Neuroscience* 9 (4): 355.

Cuesta Brey, Luis, and Kyrenia Sánchez Rodríguez. 2007. "Aspectos éticos de la experimentación con animals." *Bioética* 27: 1–3.

Cueto, Marcos. 2007. *Cold War, Deadly Fevers: Malaria Eradication in Mexico, 1955–1975*. Baltimore: John Hopkins University Press.

Currie, James. 1804. *Medical Reports, on the Effects of Water, Cold and Warm: As a Remedy in Fever and Other Diseases, Whether Applied to the Surface of the Body, Or Used Internally*. Liverpool: McCreery.

Cutler, Vanessa J. 2021. "The Science and Psychology of Beauty." In *Essential Psychiatry for the Aesthetic Practitioner*, edited by Evan Rieder and Richard Fried, 22–33. Hoboken, NJ: Wiley Blackwell.

Dalziel, George and Edward Dalziel. 1901. *The Brothers Dalziel. A Record of Fifty Years Work in Conjunction with Many of the Most Distinguished Artists of the Period 1840–1890*. London: Methuen and Co.

Danziger, Pamela. 1 September 2019. "6 Trends Shaping the Future of the $532B Beauty Business." *Forbes*.

D'Argenio, Maria Chiara. 2022. *Indigenous Plots in Twenty-First Century Latin American Cinema*. Cham: Palgrave/Springer.

Das, Plabon Kumar, Mst Ayesha Siddika, Saharia Yeasmin Asha, Suraiya Aktar, Farhadul Islam, Jahan Ara Khanam, and Md Abdur Rakib. 2019. "Investigation of Phytochemicals and Antioxidant Activities in the Leaves Methanolic Extract from Moringa Oleifera Plants Grown in Bangladesh." *Journal of Pharmacognosy and Phytochemistry* 8 (4): 2502–2508.

Datta, Shivika, Praveen C. Ramamurthy, Uttpal Anand, Simranjeet Singh, Amritpal Singh, Daljeet Singh Dhanjal, Vaishali Dhaka, et al. 2021. "Wonder or Evil?: Multifaceted Health Hazards and Health Benefits of Cannabis Sativa and its Phytochemicals." *Saudi Journal of Biological Sciences* 28 (12): 7290–7313.

Dávalos, Liliana. 2018. "The Ghosts of Development Past: Deforestation and Coca in Western Amazonia." In *The Origins of Cocaine*, edited by Paul Gootenberg and Liliana Dávalos, 19–52. London: Routledge.

David, Sara, and Carol Allan. 2018. "Midwives Influencing Community Acceptance of Family Planning to Reduce Maternal Mortality Rates in Remote Villages of Papua New Guinea Where Men are the Gatekeepers." *Women and Birth* 31: S52.

Dawson, Angela, Annette Nkowane, and Anna Whelan. 2015. "Approaches to Improving the Contribution of the Nursing and Midwifery Workforce to Increasing Universal Access to Primary Health Care for Vulnerable Populations: A Systematic Review." *Human Resources for Health* 13 (1): 1–23.

Deb Roy, Rohan. 2017. *Malarial Subjects: Empire, Medicine and Nonhumans in British India, 1820–1909.* Cambridge: Cambridge University Press.

de Guignes, Joseph. 1756. *Histoire Générale Des Huns, Des Turcs, Des Mogols, et Des Autres Tartares Occidentaux.* Volume 1. Paris: Desaint et Saillant.

de la Cruz, Martín.1552. *Libellus de Medicinalibus Indorum Herbis* [Cruz-Badiano Codex]. Translated by Juan Badiano. México.

Delumeau, Jean. 1983. *Le péché et la peur: la culpabilisation en Occident.* Paris: Fayard.

de Palafox y Mendoza, Juan. 1670. *Histoire de la conqueste de la Chine par les Tartares.* Paris: Librairie de la Reyne.

De Regt, Anouk, Matteo Montecchi, and Sarah Lord Ferguson. 2019. "A False Image of Health: How Fake News and Pseudo-facts Spread in the Health and Beauty Industry." *Journal of Product & Brand Management* 29 (2): 168–179.

Diaz Soto, Lourdes. 2000. *The Politics of Early Childhood Education.* New York, NY: Peter Lang.

Dibble, Charles, and Arthur Anderson. 1963. *Florentine Codex: General History of the Things of New Spain, Fray Bernardino de Sahagún. Book 11 – Earthly Things.* Santa Fe, NM: The School of American Research and the University of Utah.

Dickstein, Jonathan. 2021. "Sacred Cows & Chicken Manchurian: The Everyday Politics of Eating Meat in India." *Himalaya* 40 (2): 164–166.

Dini, Irene, and Sonia Laneri. 2021. "The New Challenge of Green Cosmetics: Natural Food Ingredients for Cosmetic Formulations." *Molecules* 26 (13): 3921.

Dovey, Jonathan, and Helen W. Kennedy. 2007. "From Margin to Center: Biographies of Technicity and the Construction of Hegemonic Games Culture." In *The*

Players' Realm: Studies on the Culture of Video Games and Gaming, edited by Jonas Smith, 131–153. Jefferson, NC: McFarland.

Driscoll, Catherine. 2011. *Teen Film: A Critical Introduction.* Oxford: Berg.

Drissi, Anas, Josefa Girona, Mounia Cherki, Gemma Godàs, Abdelfettah Derouiche, Mariame El Messal, Rachid Saile, et al. 2004. "Evidence of Hypolipemiant and Antioxidant Properties of Argan Oil Derived from the Argan Tree (*Argania spinosa*)." *Clinical Nutrition* 23 (5): 1159–1166.

Dupey García, Elodie, and María Luisa Vázquez de Ágredos Pascual, eds. 2019. *Painting the Skin: Pigments on Bodies and Codices in Pre-Columbian Mesoamerica.* Tucson-Mexico City: University of Arizona Press.

Durán-Martínez, Angélica. 2017. *The Politics of Drug Violence: Criminals, Cops and Politicians in Colombia and Mexico.* Oxford: Oxford University Press.

Eagle, Lynne, and Rachel Hay. 2020. "Appearances Matter: The Impact of Unattainable Idealizations of an Individual's Physical Self." *The SAGE Handbook of Marketing Ethics* 2: 169–183.

Eggerstedt, Michael, Jessica Rhee, Matthew J. Urban, Angelica Mangahas, Ryan M. Smith, and Peter C. Revenaugh. 2020. "Beauty is in the Eye of the Follower: Facial Aesthetics in the Age of Social Media." *American Journal of Otolaryngology* 41 (6): 102643.

Eimreiðin. 1 May 1914.

Einarsson, Gunnlaugur. 1938. "Finsk baðstofa tekur öllum böðum fram." *Morgunblaðið*, November 20, 1938.

Einarsson, Þorsteinn. 1 June 1945. "Þjóðskáldið Jónas Hallgrímsson og sundmennt Íslendinga." *Íþróttablaðið*.

El Abbassi, Abdelilah, Nauman Khalid, Hanaa Zbakh, and Asif Ahmad. 2014. "Physicochemical Characteristics, Nutritional Properties, and Health Benefits of Argan Oil: A Review." *Critical Reviews in Food Science and Nutrition* 54 (11): 1401–1414.

El-Bizri, Nader. 2001. "Avicenna and Essentialism." *The Review of Metaphysics* 54 (4): 753–778.

Elicina Official Site. 2020.

Elliott, Simon, Tanith Holdbrook, and Simon Brandt. 2020. "Prodrugs of New Psychoactive Substances (NPS): A New Challenge." *Journal of Forensic Sciences* 6 (3): 913–920.

El Monfalouti, Hanae, Dom Guillaume, Clément Denhez, and Zoubida Charrouf. 2010. "Therapeutic Potential of Argan Oil: A Review." *Journal of Pharmacy and Pharmacology* 62 (12): 1669–1675.

Elvin-Lewis, Memory. 2001. "Should We Be Concerned about Herbal Remedies?" *Journal of Ethnopharmacology* 75 (2–3): 141–164.

Emmart, Emily Walcott. 1935. "An Aztec Medical Treatise, The Badianus Manuscript." *Bulletin of the Institute of the History of Medicine* 3 (6): 483–506.

Emmart, Emily Walcott. 1940. *The Badianus Manuscript* (Codex Barberini, Latin 241). Baltimore: Johns Hopkins Press.

Ericson, Steven J. 2014. "The 'Matsukata Deflation' Reconsidered: Financial Stabilization and Japanese Exports in a Global Depression, 1881–85." *The Journal of Japanese Studies* 40 (1): 1–28.

Evans-Brown, Michael, and Roumen Sedefov. 2018. "Responding to New Psychoactive Substances in the European Union: Early Warning, Risk Assessment, and Control Measures." In *New Psychoactive Substances,* edited by Hans Maurer and Simon Brandt, 3–49. Cham: Springer.

Farajova, Malahat. 2011. "Gobustan: Rock Art Cultural Landscape." *Adoranten* 1: 1–26.

Farshtey, Gregory, and Daniel Lipkowitz. 2013. *Lego: Minifigure Year by Year: A Visual History.* London: DK.

Fatima, Samar, and Samreen Lodhi. 2015. "Impact of Advertisement on Buying Behaviours of the Consumers: Study of Cosmetic Industry in Karachi City." *International Journal of Management Sciences and Business Research* 4 (10): 125–137.

Feinberg, Ben. 2018. "Undiscovering the pueblo mágico: Lessons from Huautla for the psychedelic renaissance." In *Plant medicines, healing and psychedelic science,* edited by Beatriz Caiuby Labate and Clancy Cavnar, 37–54. Cham: Springer.

Ferguson, Priscilla Parkhurst. 2004. *Accounting for Taste: The Triumph of French Cuisine.* Chicago, IL: The University of Chicago Press.

Figuier, Oscar. 1840. *Mémoire sur la Composition Chimique des Escargots et sur les Préparations Pharmaceutiques dont ils sont la Base.* Montpellier: Imp. F. Gelly.

Finlay, Andrew Yule, and E. C. Coles. 1995. "The Effect of Severe Psoriasis on the Quality of Life of 369 Patients." *British Journal of Dermatology* 132 (2): 236–244.

Fischer, Bob. 2019. *The Ethics of Eating Animals: Usually Bad, Sometimes Wrong, Often Permissible.* London: Routledge.

Fish, Bruce, and Becky Burost Fish. 2002. *Angola, 1880 to the Present: Slavery, Exploitation, and Revolt.* Philadelphia: Chelsea House.

Fraser, Alistair. 2017. *Global Foodscapes.* New York: Routledge.

Friðjónsdóttir, Hólmfríður Dagný. 2020. *"Kvöl og pína" að komast ekki í sund."* RÚV Fréttir, May 17, 2020.

Fujita, Mako, Miho Yoshimura, Masatoshi Nakamura, Tatsuya Hojo, and Yoshiyuki Fukuoka. 2022. "Anaerobic Performance after 3-day Consecutive CO2-rich Cold-water Immersion in Physically Active Males." *Journal of Exercise Science and Fitness* 20 (2): 148–154.

Fulford, Kenneth William Musgrave. 1989. *Moral Theory and Medical Practice.* Cambridge: Cambridge University Press.

Gachelin, Gabriel, Paul Garner, Eliana Ferroni, Ulrich Tröhler, and Iain Chalmers. 2017. "Evaluating Cinchona Bark and Quinine for Treating and Preventing Malaria." *Journal of the Royal Society of Medicine* 110 (1): 31–40.

Gänger, Stefanie. 2020. *A Singular Remedy: Cinchona Across the Atlantic World, 1751–1820.* Cambridge: Cambridge University Press.

García-Sánchez, Liliana, Álvaro José Montiel-Jarquín, Eduardo Vázquez-Cruz, Adriana May-Salazar, Itzel Gutiérrez-Gabriel, and Jorge Loría-Castellanos. 2017. "Quality of Life in Patients with Psoriasis." *Gaceta medica de Mexico* 153 (2): 185–189.

Gates, William. 1939. *The De La Cruz – Badiano Aztec Herbal of 1552.* Translation and Commentary. Baltimore: The Maya Society.

Gentili, Valentina, Daria Bortolotti, Mascia Benedusi, Andrea Alogna, Anna Fantinati, Anna Guiotto, Giulia Turrin, et al. 2020. "HelixComplex Snail Mucus as a Potential Technology against O3 Induced Skin Damage." *Plos One* 15 (2): e0229613.

George, Daniel, Ryan Hanson, Darryl Wilkinson, and Albert Garcia-Romeu. 2021. "Ancient Roots of Today's Emerging Renaissance in Psychedelic Medicine." *Culture, Medicine, and Psychiatry*: 1–14.

George, Jamilah, Timothy I. Michaels, Jae Sevelius, and Monnica T. Williams. 2020. "The Psychedelic Renaissance and the Limitations of a White-dominant Medical Framework: A Call for Indigenous and Ethnic Minority Inclusion." *Journal of Psychedelic Studies* 4 (1): 4–15.

Gerber, Pierre J., Anne Mottet, Carolyn I. Opio, Alessandra Falcucci, and Félix Teillard. 2015. "Environmental Impacts of Beef Production: Review of Challenges and Perspectives for Durability." *Meat Science* 109: 2–12.

Gewertz, Deborah, and Frederick Errington. 2010. *Cheap Meat: Flap Food Nations in the South Pacific*. Berkeley: University of California Press.

Ghodsee, Kristen. 2007. "Potions, Lotions and Lipstick: The Gendered Consumption of Cosmetics and Perfumery in Socialist and Post-Socialist Urban Bulgaria." *Women's Studies International Forum* 30 (1): 26–39.

Giffort, Danielle. 2020. *Acid Revival: The Psychedelic Renaissance and the Quest for Medical Legitimacy*. Minneapolis: University of Minnesota Press.

Gimmel, Millie. 2008. "Reading Medicine in the Codex de la Cruz Badiano." *Journal of the History of Ideas* 69 (2): 169–192.

Gindhart, Maria. 2014. "Ethnographic Exoticism: Charles-Arthur Bourgeois's Snake Charmer." *Material Culture Review* 79: 7–23.

Ginneken, Jaap van. 2007. *Screening Difference*. Lanham, MD: Rowman and Littlefield.

Ginsburg, Faye. 2011. "Native Intelligence: A Short History of Debates on Indigenous Media and Ethnographic Film." In *Made to be Seen: Perspectives on the History of Visual Anthropology*, edited by Marcus Banks and Jay Ruby, 234–255. Chicago-London: University of Chicago Press.

Goik, Urszula, Tomasz Goik, and Izabela Załęska. 2019. "The Properties and Application of Argan Oil in Cosmetology." *European Journal of Lipid Science and Technology* 121 (4): 1800313.

Goldman, Peter. 2001. "Herbal Medicines Today and the Roots of Modern Pharmacology." *Annals of Internal Medicine* 135: 594–600.

Goldstein, Beth. 1975. "Ginseng: Its History, Dispersion, and Folk Tradition." *The American Journal of Chinese Medicine* 3 (3): 223–234.

Gómez-Dantés, Héctor, and Anne-Emanuelle Birn. 2000. "Malaria and Social Movements in Mexico: The Last 60 Years." *Parassitologia* 42 (1): 69–86.

Gomez-Flores, Ricardo, et al. 2000. "Immunoenhancing Properties of Plantago Major Leaf Extract." *Phytotherapy Research: An International Journal Devoted to Pharmacological and Toxicological Evaluation of Natural Product Derivatives* 14 (8): 617–622.

González-Minero, Francisco José, and Luis Bravo-Díaz. 2018. "The Use of Plants in Skin-care Products, Cosmetics and Fragrances: Past and Present." *Cosmetics* 5 (3): 50.

Gonzalez Rodriguez, Milton Fernando. 2020. "Lego® Minifigures: Reflections of Human Diversity through the Materialization of Archetypes." *Denkste Puppe* 3 (1.2): 45–51.

Gonzalez Rodriguez, Milton Fernando. 2022. *Indigeneity in Latin American Cinema*. London-New York: Bloomsbury.

Goosens, William. 1980. "Values, Health, and Medicine." *Philosophy of Science* 47 (1): 100–115.

Graham, Harvey. 1951. *Eternal Eve: The History of Gynaecology & Obstetrics*. Garden City: Doubleday & Co.

Granziera, Patrizia. 2001. "Concept of the Garden in Pre-Hispanic Mexico." *Garden History* 29 (2): 185–213.

Gross, Larry. 2002. "Minorities, Majorities and the Media." In *Media, Ritual, and Identity*, edited by Tamar Liebes, James Curran, and Elihu Katz, 71–84. London: Routledge.

Gruber, Thomas. 1993. "A Translation Approach to Portable Ontology Specifications." *Knowledge Acquisition* 5 (2): 199–220.

Grund, Jean-Paul, and Joost J. Breeksema. 2017. "Drug policy in the Netherlands." In *European Drug Policies: The Ways of Reform*, edited by Renauld Colson and Henri Bergeron, 128–148. London: Routledge.

Gualda, Dulce Maria Rosa, Nádia Zanon Narchi, and Edemilson Antunes De Campos. 2012. "Strengthening Midwifery in Brazil: Education, Regulation and Professional Association of Midwives." *Midwifery* 29 (10): 1077–1081.

Guerra-Doce, Elisa. 2015. "Psychoactive Substances in Prehistoric Times: Examining the Archaeological Evidence." *Time and Mind* 8 (1): 91–112.

Guerrero, David. 2010. "On a Naturalist Theory of Health: A Critique." *Studies in History and Philosophy of Science Part C: Studies in History and Philosophy of Biological and Biomedical Sciences* 41 (3): 272–278.

Guerrini, Anita. 2003. *Experimenting with Humans and Animals: From Galen to Animal Rights*. Baltimore: John Hopkins University Press.

Guillaume, Dom, and Zoubida Charrouf. 2011. "Argan Oil." *Alternative Medicine Review* 16 (3): 275–276.

Gullone, Eleonora. 2017. "Why Eating Animals is not Good for Us." *Journal of Animal Ethics* 7 (1): 31–62.

Gunnarsdottir, María J., Sigurdur M. Garðarsson, Gunnar St. Jónsson, and Jamie Bartram. 2016. "Chemical Quality and Regulatory Compliance of Drinking Water in Iceland." *International Journal of Hygiene and Environmental Health* 8: 724–733.

Gutwald, Rebecca. 2017. "Girl, LEGO® Friends is not Your Friend! Does LEGO® Construct Gender Stereotypes?" In *LEGO® and Philosophy*, edited by Sondra Bacharach and Roy Cook, 103–112. London: Wiley Backwell.

Gynther, Bent. 2001. *Assiliartalersugaq*. Nuuk: Atuakkiorfik Illinniusiorfik.

Hailwood, Mark, Torsten Kolind, Betsy Thom, and Geoffrey Hunt. 2016. "Historical Perspectives." In *The Sage Handbook of Drug and Alcohol Studies*, 9–29. London: Sage.

Hall, Marcus, and Dan Tamïr. 2022. *Mosquitopia*. New York: Routledge.

Hall, Wayne, Eva Hoch, and Valentina Lorenzetti. 2019. "Cannabis Use and Mental Health: Risks and Benefits." *European Archives of Psychiatry and Clinical Neuroscience* 269 (1): 1–3.

Hallgrímsson, Jónas. 1836. *Sund-reglur próf. Nachtegalls, auknar og lagaðar e. Íslanns þörfum*. Copenhagen: P.N. Jörgensen.

Hamati-Ataya, Inanna. 2022. "Globality in Deep Time: Ontological Frames and Repertoires of Historicisation." Paper presented at the Graduate Institute Geneva, 24 March 2022.

Hamelin, Nicolas, Amina Mokannef, and Ayantunji Gbadamosi. 2018. "Colour Cosmetics Consumption Among Moroccan Women: Examining the Nexus of Attitudes, Religion and the Media." *International Journal of Consumer Studies* 42 (6): 755–767.

Hamid ElKhoreiby, Inas Abdel. 2021. "The Social Comparison Theory in the Context of Cosmetic Plastic Surgery Advertising: Predictors and Consequences of their Impact on Women." لاصتالاو مالعالا ثوحبل ةيبرعلا ةلجملا n. 34: 2–35.

Han, Dong-Woon, and Tae-Hyung Yoon. 2005. "Current Circumstance and Issues in Interface between Western Medicine and Traditional Korean Medicine in Korea: What are Health Policy Options for a New Integrative Health System?" *Journal of Society of Preventive Korean Medicine* 9 (2): 43–58.

Han, Gil Soo. 1997. "The Rise of Western Medicine and Revival of Traditional Medicine in Korea: A Brief History." *Korean Studies* 21 (1): 96–121.

Hansen, Keld. 2009. *Nuussuarmiut – Hunting Families on the Big Headland: Demography, Subsistence and Material Culture in Nuussuaq, Upernavik, Northwest Greenland*. Copenhagen: Museum Tusculanum Press, University of Copenhagen.

Hanson, Debra. 2014. "Orientalism Today: Revisions and Remakings." *Tasmeem* 1: 5.

Harris, Eric. 2008. "Ethnobryology: Traditional Uses and Folk Classification of Bryophytes." *The Bryologist* 111 (2): 169–217.

Hasan, Md Mahadi, Iffat-Ara Sharmeen, Yasir Anwar, Hesham F. Alharby, Mirza Hasanuzzaman, Abdulrahaman S. Hajar, and Khalid Rehman Hakeem. 2019. "Evidence-based Assessment of Moringa oleifera used for the Treatment of Human Ailments." *Plant and Human Health* 2: 121–137. Cham: Springer.

Hasanudin, Khairunnisa, Puziah Hashim, and Shuhaimi Mustafa. 2012. "Corn Silk (*Stigma maydis*) in Healthcare: A Phytochemical and Pharmacological Review." *Molecules* 17 (8): 9697–9715.

Hastrup, Kirsten. 2008. "Icelandic Topography and the Sense of Identity." In *Nordic Landscapes*, edited by Michael Jones and Kenneth Olwig, 53–76. Minneapolis: University of Minnesota Press.

Haug, Wolfgang Fritz. 1986 (1971). *Critique of Commodity Aesthetics: Appearance, Sexual and Advertising in Capitalist Society*. Translated by Robert Bock. Cambridge: Polity.

Hayden, Cori. 2005. "Bioprospecting's Representational Dilemma." *Science as Culture* 14 (2): 185–200.

Heaton, Matthew. 2018. "Health and Medicine in Colonial Society." In *The Palgrave Handbook of African Colonial and Postcolonial History*, edited by Martin Shanguhyia and Toyin Falola, 303–317. New York, NY: Palgrave Macmillan.

Hedhili, Amel, Samuel Lubbers, Elias Bou-Maroun, Francine Griffon, Babatope Ebenezer Akinyemi, Florence Husson, and Dominique Valentin. 2021. "Moringa Oleifera Supplemented Biscuits: Nutritional Values and Consumer Segmentation." *South African Journal of Botany* 138: 406–414.

Heinonen, Ilkka, and Jari Laukkanen. 2018. "Effects of Heat and Cold on Health, with Special Reference to Finnish Sauna Bathing." *American Journal of Physiology Regulatory, Integrative and Comparative Physiology* 314 (5): R629–R638.

Hendy, Katherine. 2021. "What Can the Chemical Hold?: The Politics of Efficacy in the Psychedelic Renaissance." *Culture, Medicine, and Psychiatry*: 1–22.

Hill, Mary, Azin Kheirandish Pishkenari, Taylor Braunberger, April Armstrong, and Cory Dunnick. 2016. "Recent Trends in Disease Severity and Quality of Life Instruments for Patients with Atopic Dermatitis: A Systematic Review." *Journal of the American Academy of Dermatology* 75 (5): 906–917.

Hines, Edgar, and George Brown. 1932. "A Standard Stimulant for Measuring Vasomotor Reactions: Its Application in the Study of Hypertension." *Proceedings of the Staff Meetings of the Mayo Clinic* 7: 332–325.

Hinojosa, Servando. 2004. "Authorizing Tradition: Vectors of Contention in Highland Maya Midwifery." *Social Science and Medicine* 59 (3): 637–651.

Hohenauer, Erich, Tom Deliens, Peter Clarys, and Ron Clijsen. 2019. "Perfusion of the skin's microcirculation after cold-water immersion (10 C) and partial-body cryotherapy (– 135 C)." *Skin Research and Technology* 25 (5): 677–682.

Hokkanen, Markku. 2017. *Medicine, Mobility and the Empire*. Manchester: Manchester University Press.

Hölker, Sarah, Marie von Meyer-Höfer, and Achim Spiller. 2019. "Animal Ethics and Eating Animals: Consumer Segmentation Based on Domain-specific Values." *Sustainability* 11 (14): 3907.

Holm, Jesper, Tove Agner, Maja-Lisa Clausen, and Simon Francis Thomsen. 2016. "Quality of Life and Disease Severity in Patients with Atopic Dermatitis." *Journal of the European Academy of Dermatology and Venereology* 30 (10): 1760–1767.

Holoyda, Brian. 2020. "The Psychedelic Renaissance and Its Forensic Implications." *The Journal of the American Academy of Psychiatry and the Law* 48 (1): 87–97.

Horn, Armin, Arnaud Pascal, Isidora Lončarević, Raíssa Volpatto Marques, Yi Lu, Sissi Miguel, Frederic Bourgaud, et al. 2021. "Natural Products from Bryophytes: From Basic Biology to Biotechnological Applications." *Critical Reviews in Plant Sciences* 40 (3): 191–217.

Hu, Meibian, Zhijie Yu, Jiaolong Wang, Wenxiang Fan, Yujie Liu, Jianghua Li, He Xiao, Yongchuan Li, Wei Peng, and Chunjie Wu. 2017. "Traditional Uses, Origins, Chemistry and Pharmacology of *Bombyx batryticatus*: A Review." *Molecules* 22 (10): 1779.

Huart, Louis. 10 March 1851. "Le vein de ginseng." *Le Charivari*.

Huezo, Alexander. 2019. "Contested Natures: Coca, the War on Drugs, and Ecologies of Difference in Colombia's Afro-Pacific." *Journal of Political Ecology* 26 (1): 305–322.

Huggan, Graham, and Helen Tiffin. 2015. *Postcolonial Ecocriticism: Literature, Animals, Environment.* London: Routledge.

Hurtienne, Jörn, Christian Stößel, and Katharina Weber. 2009. "Sad Is Heavy and Happy Is Light: Population Stereotypes of Tangible Object Attributes." In *Proceedings of the 3rd International Conference on Tangible and Embedded Interaction*, 61–68. Cambridge, UK.

Hussan, Farida, Adila Sofea Mansor, Siti Nazihahasma Hassan, Tengku Nor Effendy Kamaruddin, Tg Nurul Tasnim, Siti Balkis Budin, and Faizah Othman. 2015. "Anti-inflammatory Property of Plantago Major Leaf Extract Reduces the Inflammatory Reaction in Experimental Acetaminophen-induced Liver Injury." *Evidence-Based Complementary and Alternative Medicine* 2015: 347861.

Huttunen, Pirkko, Leena Kokko, and Virpi Ylijukuri. 2004. "Winter Swimming Improves General Well-being." *International Journal of Circumpolar Health* 63 (2): 140–144.

Huy, Dinh Tran Ngoc. 2021. "The Impact of Pro-environmental Beliefs and Personal Norms on Green Cosmetics Purchase Intention: A Study of Gen Z in Vietnam." *Revista Geintec- Gestão, Inovação e Tecnologias* 1 (2): 1748–1763.

Ikpeazu, Victor O., Eziuche A. Ugbogu, Okezie Emmanuel, Chikezie Uche-Ikonne, Benedict Okoro, and Jennifer Nnaemeka. 2018. "Evaluation of the Safety of Oral Intake of Aqueous Extract of *Stigma Maydis* (corn silk) in Rats." *Acta Scientiarum Polonorum Technologia Alimentaria* 17 (4): 387–397.

Ingarden, Roman Witold. 1964. *Der Streit urn die Existenz der Welt.* Vol. 1: Existentialontologie. Tübingen: Niemeyer.

Ísafold. 14 September 1889.

Ísafold. 7 April 1927.

Ishikawa, Hideki, Masaki Matsushima, Masami Nagashima, and Akiko Osuga. 1992. "Screening of Children with Arrhythmias for Arrhythmia Development during Diving and Swimming: Face Immersion as a Substitute for Diving and Exercise Stress Testing as a Substitute for Swimming." *Japanese Circulation Journal* 56 (9): 881–890.

Iversen, Leslie. 2005. "Long-term Effects of Exposure to Cannabis." *Current Opinion in Pharmacology* 5 (1): 69–72.

Jakobsen, Kirsten, and Katrine Vissing. 2011. *Min første røde ordbog*. Copenhagen: Gyldendal.

Janet, Pierre. 1901. "La maladie du scrupule ou l'aboulie délirante: le contenu des obsessions." *Revue Philosophique de La France et de l'Étranger* 51: 337–359.

Jay, Mike. 2019. *Mescaline: A Global History of the First Psychedelic.* Llandysul: Yale University Press.

Jayapandian, Catherine, Chien-Hung Chen, Aman Dabir, Samden Lhatoo, Guo-Qiang Zhang, and Satya S. Sahoo. "Domain ontology as conceptual model for big data management: application in biomedical informatics." In *International Conference on Conceptual Modeling*, 144–157. Springer, Cham.

Jeacle, Ingrid. 2006. "Face Facts: Accounting, Feminism and the Business of Beauty." *Critical Perspectives on Accounting* 17 (1): 87–108.

Jenkins, Gwynne. 2001. "Changing Roles and Identities of Midwives in Rural Costa Rica." *Medical Anthropology* 20 (4): 409–444.

Jenkins, Henry. 1998. "Introduction: Childhood Innocence and Other Modern Myths." In *The Children's Culture Reader*, edited by Henry Jenkins, 1–40. New York, NY: New York University Press.

Jeong, Yun Hee, You-Chang Oh, Won-Kyung Cho, Hye Jin Yang, and Jin Yeul Ma. 2017. "*Maydis Stigma* Elicits Analgesia and Blocks Edema in Mice and Inhibits Inflammation in Macrophages." *The American Journal of Chinese Medicine* 45 (7): 1477–1496.

Jinsheng, Zheng, and 鄭金生. 2018. "Observational Drawing and Fine Art in Chinese Materia Medica Illustration." In *Imagining Chinese Medicine*, edited by Vivienne Lo, 羅維前, Penelope Barrett, David Dear, Lu Di, 蘆笛, Lois Reynolds, Dolly Yang, and 楊德秀, 151–160. Leiden: Brill.

Jóhannesson, Torfi. 2010. *Agriculture in Iceland: Conditions and Characteristics.* Reykjavik/Hvanneyri: The Agricultural University of Iceland.

Johnson, Derek. 2014. "Figuring Identity: Media Licensing and the Racialization of LEGO Bodies." *International Journal of Cultural Studies* 17 (4): 307–325.

Jónsson, Örn Daníel. 2013. "Heiti potturinn - vinsælasti samkomustaður landsins." *Tímarti Máls og menningar* 2: 120–125.

Jónsson, Örn Daníel, and Ólafur Rastrick. 2017. "Enjoying the Outdoor Pool in a Cold Climate: Appropriate Technology, Utilisation of Geothermal Resources and the Socialisation of Everyday Practices in Iceland." *Geothermal Energy* 5 (1): 1–14.

Jordanova, Ludmilla. 1995. "The Social Construction of Medical Knowledge." *Social History of Medicine* 8 (3): 361–381.

Jordanova, Ludmilla. 2019. "Reflection: Pictures of Health?" In *Health: A History*, edited by Peter Adamson, 246–250. Oxford: Oxford University Press.

Joshi, Ashish, Rinzin Wangmo, and Chioma Amadi. 2017. "Blogs as Channels for Disseminating Health Technology Innovations." *Healthcare Informatics Research* 23 (3): 208–217.

Joung, Hyunchae, Bobae Kim, Hyunjoon Park, Kyuyeon Lee, Hee-Hoon Kim, Ho-Cheol Sim, Hyun-Jin Do, Chang-Kee Hyun, and Myoung-Sool Do. 2017. "Fermented Moringa Oleifera Decreases Hepatic Adiposity and Ameliorates Glucose Intolerance in High-Fat Diet-Induced Obese Mice." *Journal of Medicinal Food* 20 (5): 439–447.

Juhász, Margit, Melissa Levin, and Ellen Marmur. 2018. "The Use of Natural Ingredients in Innovative Korean Cosmeceuticals." *Journal of Cosmetic Dermatology* 17 (3): 305–312.

Jun, Heo. 1613. *Donguibogam, Principles and Practice of Eastern Medicine* (동의보감(東醫寶鑑). English Translation of the Donguibogam -Korea Institute of Oriental Medicine.

Jung, Jaehee. 2018. "Young Women's Perceptions of Traditional and Contemporary Female Beauty Ideals in China." *Family and Consumer Sciences Research Journal* 47 (1): 56–72.

Jurásek, Bronislav, Ivan Čmelo, Jan Svoboda, Jan Čejka, Daniel Svozil, and Martin Kuchař. 2021. "New Psychoactive Substances on Dark Web Markets: From Deal Solicitation to Forensic Analysis of Purchased Substances." *Drug Testing and Analysis* 13 (1): 156–168.

Kahn, Miriam. 1998. "'Men are taro' (they cannot be rice): Political Aspects of Food Choices in Wamira, Papua New Guinea." In *Food and Gender: Identity and Power*, edited by Carole M. Counihan and Steven L. Kaplan, 30–46. Amsteldijk: Harwood.

Kandall, Stephen. 2010. "Women and Drug Addiction: A Historical Perspective." *Journal of Addictive Diseases* 29 (2): 117–126.

Kang, Youngmi, Won Ju Hwang, and Ji Sun Choi. 2019. "A Concept Analysis of Traditional Korean (Hanbang) Nursing." *International Journal of Nursing Knowledge* 30 (1): 4–11.

Kartawinata, Budi Rustandi, Dyah Maharani, Mahir Pradana, and Hilda Maulida Amani. 2020. "The Role of Customer Attitude in Mediating the Effect of Green Marketing Mix on Green Product Purchase Intention in Love Beauty and Planet Products in Indonesia." *Proceedings of the International Conference on Industrial Engineering and Operations Management* 1: 3023–3033.

Kelly, John, Abuzar Baker, Mohamed Babiker, Lisa Burke, Christine Brennan, and Veronica O'Keane. 2019. "The Psychedelic Renaissance: The Next Trip for Psychiatry?" *Irish Journal of Psychological Medicine*: 1–5. doi:10.1017/ipm.2019.39.

Kenny, Glenn, Prud'homme Denis, Card Eric Proulx, and Gordon Giesbrecht. 1999. "The Effect of Dynamic Exercise on Resting Cold Thermoregulatory Responses Measured During Water Immersion." *European Journal of Applied Physiology and Occupational Physiology* 79 (6): 495–499.

Keshet, Yael. 2009. "The Untenable Boundaries of Biomedical Knowledge: Epistemologies and Rhetoric Strategies in the Debate over Evaluating Complementary and Alternative Medicine." *Health* 13 (2): 131–155.

Kettemann, Bernhard. 2017. "Orientalism/Occidentalism." *The Polyphony of English Studies: A Festschrift for Allan James* 26: 177.

Kevles, Daniel. 2020. *Heirloom Fruits of America: Selections from the USDA Pomological Watercolor Collection.* Berkeley: Heyday Press.

Khaltaev, Nikolai, Umberto Solimene, Federico Vitale, and Alessandro Zanasi. 2020. "Balneotherapy and Hydrotherapy in Chronic Respiratory Disease." *Journal of Thoracic Disease* 12 (8): 4459–4468.

Kharbach, Mourad, Huiwen Yu, Rabie Kamal, Issam Barra, Ilias Marmouzi, Yahia Cherrah, Katim Alaoui, Abdelaziz Bouklouze, and Yvan Vander Heyden. 2021. "New Insights into the Argan Oil Categories Characterization: Chemical Descriptors, FTIR Fingerprints, and Chemometric Approaches." *Talanta* 225: 122073.

Kim, Beom Joon, Yeon A. No, Yonghee Lee, Myung Nam Kim, Chang Kwon Hong, Kwang Ho Yoo, Yong Min Kim, Jung Hyun Hwang, and Su Yeon Kong. 2015. "Use of Cream Containing Mucus Secreted by Snails has an Anti-Aging Effect on Skin." *Korean Journal of Dermatology* 53 (6): 430–436.

Kim, Chung-Il. 2008. 칠레산 달팽이 크림 인기…'피부재생 탁월' 입소문 – 매일경제.

Kimmel, Michael. 2001. "Masculinities and Femininities." In *International Encyclopedia of the Social & Behavioral Sciences*, 9318–9321. London: Elsevier.

Kingma, Elselijn. 2019. "Contemporary Accounts of Health." In *Health: A History*, edited by Peter Adamson, 289–318. Oxford: Oxford University Press.

Kirby, David. 2010. *Animal Factory: The Looming Threat of Industrial Pig, Dairy, and Poultry Farms to Humans and the Environment*. New York: St. Martin's Press.

Kirchfeld, Friedhelm, and Wade Boyle. 1994. *Nature Doctors. Pioneers in Naturopathic Medicine*. Portland: NCNM Press.

Kitāb al-Diryāq (كتاب الدرياق.)/ *Book of Antidotes*. 1198–1199.

Kitton, Frederic George. 1883. *John Leech, Artist and Humorist: A Biographical Sketch*. London: G. Redway.

Klein, Shana. 2020. *The Fruits of Empire*. Oakland: University of California Press.

Kler, Joseph. 1969. *Medicine on Stamps*. New York: Minkus Publications.

Knechtle, Beat, Zbigniew Waśkiewicz, Caio Victor Sousa, Lee Hill, and Pantelis T. Nikolaidis. 2020. "Cold Water Swimming-Benefits and Risks: A Narrative Review." *International Journal of Environmental Research and Public Health* 17 (23): 8984.

Knight, Christine. 2008. "'The Food Nature Intended You to Eat': Nutritional Primitivism in Low-carbohydrate Diet Discourse." PhD diss., University of Adelaide.

Konadu, Kwasi. 2008. "Medicine and Anthropology in Twentieth Century Africa: Akan Medicine and Encounters with (Medical) Anthropology." *African Studies Quarterly* 10: 45–69.

Koszorú, Kamilla, Júlia Borza, László Gulácsi, and Miklós Sárdy. 2019. "Quality of Life in Patients with Atopic Dermatitis." *Cutis* 104 (3): 174–177.

Kou, Xianjuan, Biao Li, Julia B. Olayanju, Justin M. Drake, and Ning Chen. 2018. "Nutraceutical or Pharmacological Potential of Moringa Oleifera Lam." *Nutrients* 10 (3): 343.

Koukouraki, Pelagia, Alexandros Tsoupras, Georgios Sotiroudis, Constantinos A. Demopoulos, and Theodore G. Sotiroudis. 2020. "Antithrombotic Properties of Spirulina Extracts against Platelet-activating Factor and Thrombin." *Food Bioscience* 37: 100686.

Kreps, Gary L. 2001. "The Evolution and Advancement of Health Communication Inquiry." *Annals of the International Communication Association* 24 (1): 231–253.

Kuhn, Thomas. 1962. *The Structure of Scientific Revolutions*. Chicago: University of Chicago Press.

Kuld, Jóhannes J. E. 1939. *Berklavarnablaðið*. Reykjavik: Sjálfsvörn, félag berklasjúklinga, Kristneshæli (1939–1940).

Kunle, Oluyemisi Folashade, Henry Omoregie Egharevba, and Peter Ochogu Ahmadu. 2012. "Standardization of Herbal Medicines: A Review." *International Journal of Biodiversity and Conservation* 4 (3): 101–112.

Kwak, Yeunhee and Yoonjung Kim. 2017. "Health-related Quality of Life and Mental Health of Adults with Atopic Dermatitis." *Archives of Psychiatric Nursing* 31 (5): 516–521.

La Démocratie. 1932–1936.

LaFoy, Jo, and Elizabeth A. Geden. 1989. "Postepisiotomy Pain: Warm Versus Cold Sitz Bath." *Journal of Obstetric, Gynecologic, and Neonatal Nursing* 18 (5): 399–403.

Lamy, Jean-Baptiste. 2016. "Ontology-oriented Programming for Biomedical Informatics." In *Transforming Healthcare with the Internet of Things*, edited by Jacob Hofdijk, Brigitte Séroussi, Christian Lovis, Floor Sieverink, F. Ehrler, and Adrien Ugon, 64–68. Amsterdam: IOS Press.

Lang, Jacek. 2015. *Ilustrowany słownik: angielsko-polski*. Poznań: Publicat S.A.

Lankow, Jason, Josh Ritchie, and Ross Crooks. 2012. *Infographics: The Power of Visual Storytelling*. Hoboken, NJ: John Wiley & Sons.

Laqueur, Hannah, Ariadne Rivera-Aguirre, Aaron Shev, Alvaro Castillo-Carniglia, Kara E. Rudolph, Jessica Ramirez, Silvia S. Martins, and Magdalena Cerdá. 2020. "The Impact of Cannabis Legalization in Uruguay on Adolescent Cannabis Use." *International Journal of Drug Policy* 80: 102748.

Larrère, Raphaël. 2002. "Éthique et expérimentation animale." *Nature Sciences Sociétés* 10 (1): 24–32.

Laukötter, Anja. 2016. "How Films Entered the Classroom." *Osiris* 31 (1): 181–200.

Laurance, P. Roberts. 1976. *A Dictionary of Japanese Artists*. New York: Weatherhill.

Lbova, Liudmila. 2021. "The Siberian Paleolithic Site of Mal'ta: A Unique Source for the Study of Childhood Archaeology." *Evolutionary Human Sciences* 3: e9.

L'Œuvre. 1935–1937.

Le Courrier français. 4 May 1832.

LeBlanc, Jacques, John Arthur Hildes, and O. Héroux. 1960. "Tolerance of Gaspé Fishermen to Cold Water." *Journal of Applied Physiology* 15 (6): 1031–1034.

Lee, Chang Ho, and Jong-Hoon Kim. 2014. "A Review on the Medicinal Potentials of Ginseng and Ginsenosides on Cardiovascular Diseases." *Journal of Ginseng Research* 38 (3): 161–166.

Lee, Hye-Min. 2016. "Louis XIV's Ginseng: Shaping of Knowledge on an Herbal Medicine in the Late 17th and the Early 18th Century France." *Uisahak* 25 (1): 111–145.

Lee, So-Rim. 2018. "Performing the Self: Cosmetic Surgery and the Political Economy of Beauty in Korea." PhD diss., Stanford University.

Leerssen, Joep. 2007. "Imagology: History and Method." In *Imagology: The Cultural Construction and Literary Representation of National Characters*, edited by Manfred Beller and Joep Leerssen, 17–32. Amsterdam: Rodopi.

Lego Official Site. 2021.

Le Journal. 1932–1936.

Le Matin. 1932–1936.

Leonardi, Fabio. 2018. "The Definition of Health: Towards New Perspectives." *International Journal of Health Services* 48 (4): 735–748.

Le Tell. 24 June 1933.

Le Tintamarre. 6 April 1851.

Lev, Efraim. 2003. "Traditional Healing with Animals (Zootherapy): Medieval to Present-day Levantine Practice." *Journal of Ethnopharmacology* 85 (1): 107–118.

Levinas, Emanuel. 1996. "Is Ontology Fundamental?" In *Basic Philosophical Writings*, edited by Emanuel Levinas, 1–10. Bloomington: Indiana University Press.

Liblub, Sudjit, Lyn Gum, and Maryam Bazargan. 2020. "How do Pregnant Women Perceive the Role of the Midwife in Thailand? A Descriptive Study." *Journal of Asian Midwives* 7 (2): 33–47.

Lightman, Bernard. 2007. *Victorian Popularizers of Science: Designing Nature for New Audiences*. Chicago and London: The University of Chicago Press.

Lintner, Bertil. 2019. *Burma in Revolt: Opium and Insurgency since 1948*. London: Routledge.

Liobikienė, Genovaitė, and Jurga Bernatonienė. 2017. "Why Determinants of Green Purchase cannot be Treated Equally? The Case of Green Cosmetics: Literature Review." *Journal of Cleaner Production* 162: 109–120.

Livingstone, Sydney, et al. 1978. "Effect of Local Cold Stress on Peripheral Temperatures of Inuit, Oriental, and Caucasian Subjects." *Canadian Journal of Physiology and Pharmacology* 56 (5): 877–881.

López-Agüero, Lucía, and Anna María Stella. 2007. "Aesthetic Dermatology through the Time." *Revista Argentina de Dermatología* 88: 227–233.

López Ridaura, Cecilia. 2015. "De la mandrágora al peyote. Plantas brujeriles en España y América." In *Las minorías: Ciencia y religión, magia y superstición en España y América (siglos XV al XVII)*, edited by Rica Amrán, 52–62. Santa Barbara, CA: eHumanista.

Loyer, Jessica, and Christine Knight. 2018. "Selling the 'Inca superfood': Nutritional Primitivism in Superfoods Books and Maca Marketing." *Food, Culture & Society* 21 (4): 449–467.

Lu, Donna. 2021. "'Psychedelics Renaissance': New Wave of Research Puts Hallucinogenics Forward to Treat Mental Health." *The Guardian*, September 26, 2021.

Lutsky, Irving, Margaret Hopwood, Stephen E. Abram, James M. Cerletty, Raymond G. Hoffman, and John P. Kampine. 1994. "Use of Psychoactive Substances in Three Medical Specialties: Anaesthesia, Medicine and Surgery." *Canadian Journal of Anaesthesia* 41 (7): 561–567.

Lv, Xinmiao, Siyu Zhao, Zhangchi Ning, Honglian Zeng, Yisong Shu, Ou Tao, Cheng Xiao, Cheng Lu, and Yuanyan Liu. 2015. "Citrus Fruits as a Treasure Trove of Active Natural Metabolites that Potentially Provide Benefits for Human Health." *Chemistry Central Journal* 9: 68.

Ma, Eun Jeong. 2010. "The Medicine Cabinet: Korean Medicine under Dispute." *East Asian Science, Technology and Society: An International Journal* 4 (3): 367–382.

Madan, Aarti Smith. 2019. "Women's Street Artivism in India and Brazil: Shilo Shiv Suleman's Pan-indigenous Environmental Movement." In *Routledge Handbook of Ecocriticism and Environmental Communication*, edited by Scott Slovic, Swarnalatha Rangarajan, and Vidya Sarveswaran, 314–325. New York-London: Routledge.

Madden, Raymond. 2017. *Being Ethnographic*. London: Sage.

Madras, Bertha. 2016. "The Growing Problem of New Psychoactive Substances (NPS)." In *Neuropharmacology of New Psychoactive Substances (NPS)*, edited by Michael H. Baumann, Richard A. Glennon, and Jenny L. Wiley, 1–18. Cham: Springer.

Mahuika, Nēpia. 2019. *Rethinking Oral History and Tradition: An Indigenous Perspective*. New York: Oxford University Press.

Mäkel, Annelijn, Frans Folkvord, and Paul Nelissen. 2021. "Het promoten van gezonde voeding met behulp van vlogs." *Tijdschrift voor Communicatiewetenschap* 49 (2): 127–165.

Mangal, Sudipto, Moumita Ray, Sakshar Saha, Shubham Paul, and Himangshu S. Maji. 2021. "Perception Regarding Selection and Use of Skincare Products and the Impact of Advertisement: A Questionnaire-Based Randomized Survey." *Egyptian Pharmaceutical Journal* 20 (3): 173.

Mansfield, David. 2016. *A State Built on Sand: How Opium Undermined Afghanistan*. New York: Oxford University Press.

Mantoni, Teit, Bo Belhage, Lars Pedersen, and Frank Pott. 2007. "Reduced Cerebral Perfusion on Sudden Immersion in Ice Water: A Possible Cause of Drowning." *Aviation, Space, and Environmental Medicine* 78 (4): 374–376.

Marchant, Louis. 1902. "L'escargot dans la cuisine, la thérapeutique, l'art et la literature." *Bulletin 21 de la Société syndicale des pharmaciens de la Côte-d'or*.

de Maret, Pierre. 2016. "Tea Party Toys? Classical Kisalian Grave Goods from the Upemba (Democratic Republic of Congo)." *Journal of African Archaeology* 14 (1): 19–32.

Margócsy, Dániel. 2014. *Commercial Visions: Science, Trade, and Visual Culture in the Dutch Golden Age*. Chicago: University of Chicago Press.

Margolis, Joseph. 1976. "The Concept of Disease." *Journal of Medicine and Philosophy* 1 (3): 238–255.

Maris, Cees. 2018. "Consument in narco-staat. Is drugsgebruik wel normaal?" *Filosofie & Praktijk* 2: 62–68.

Marko, Sabovljević, Bijelović Aneta, and Grubišić Dragoljub. 2001. "Bryophytes as a Potential Source of Medicinal Compounds." *Pregl Rev* 21 (1): 17–29.

Marsh, Jackie, and Julia C. Bishop. 2013. *Changing Play: Play, Media and Commercial Culture from the 1950s to the Present Day*. Berkshire: McGrawHill.

Martuccelli, Danilo. 2016. "L'innovation, le nouvel imaginaire du changement." *Quaderni* 91: 33–45.

Mateus Mora, Angélica María. 2012. *L'Indien: images et conflits*. Paris: L'Harmattan.

Matic, Ivana, Arianna Guidi, Maurice Kenzo, Maurizio Mattei, and Andrea Galgani. 2018. "Investigation of Medicinal Plants Traditionally used as Dietary Supplements: A Review on *Moringa Oleifera*." *Journal of Public Health in Africa* 9 (3): 841.

Matić, Matea, and Barbara Puh. 2016. "Consumers' Purchase Intentions Towards Natural Cosmetics." *Ekonomski vjesnik/Econviews-Review of Contemporary Business, Entrepreneurship and Economic Issues* 29 (1): 53–64.

Mbembe, Achille. 2019. *Necropolitics*. Durham: Duke University Press.

Meagher, Kate. 2019. "Working in Chains: African Informal Workers and Global Value Chains." *Agrarian South: Journal of Political Economy* 8 (1–2): 64–92.

Mehdinezhad, Naeim, Naheed Aryaeian, Mohammadreza Vafa, Atoosa Saeedpour, Abdolali Ebrahimi, Tofigh Mobaderi, Reza Fahimi, and Zohreh Sajadi Hezaveh. 2021. "Effect of Spirulina and Chlorella alone and Combined on the Healing Process of Diabetic Wounds: An Experimental Model of Diabetic Rats." *Journal of Diabetes & Metabolic Disorders* 1 (1): 161–169.

Meireles, Diana, João Gomes, Lara Lopes, Mariana Hinzmann, and Jorge Machado. 2020. "A Review of Properties, Nutritional and Pharmaceutical Applications of *Moringa Oleifera*: Integrative Approach on Conventional and Traditional Asian Medicine." *Advances in Traditional Medicine* 20: 1–21.

Mena, Paul. 2021. "Reducing Misperceptions through News Stories with Data Visualization: The Role of Readers' Prior Knowledge and Prior Beliefs." *Journalism* doi.org/10.1177/14648849211028762 62.

Merriam Webster Online Dictionary. 2021.

Ministerio de Salud Pública y Asistencia Social. 2015. *Política Nacional de Comadronas de los Cuatro Pueblos de Guatemala 2015–2025.* Ciudad de Guatemala: Gobierno de Guatemala, Ministerio de Salud Pública y Asistencia Social.

Mintz, Sidney, and Christine Du Bois. 2002. "The Anthropology of Food and Eating." *Annual Review of Anthropology* 3 (1): 99–119.

Miranda, Tatiana Mota, Maria Christina de Mello Amorozo, José Sílvio Govone, and Daniela Mota Miranda. 2007. "The Influence of Visual Stimuli in Ethnobotanical Data Collection Using the Listing Task Method." *Field Methods* 19 (1): 76–86.

Mirzoeff, Nicholas. 2009. "The Sea and the Land: Biopower and Visuality from Slavery to Katrina." *Culture, Theory & Critique* 50 (2–3): 289–305.

Mirzoeff, Nicholas. 2014. "Visualizing the Anthropocene." *Public Culture* 26 (2): 213–232.

Mohanty, Monalisa, Samita Mohanty, Sanat Kumar Bhuyan, and Ruchi Bhuyan. 2021. "Phytoperspective of Moringa oleifera for Oral Health Care: An Innovative Ethnomedicinal Approach." *Phytotherapy Research* 35 (3): 1345–1357.

Monani, Salma, and Joni Adamson. 2017. *Ecocriticism and Indigenous Studies: Conversations from Earth to Cosmos.* New York-London: Routledge.

Morganti, Pierfrancesco, Gianluca Morganti, Alessandro Gagliardini, and Alka Lohani. 2021. "From Cosmetics to Innovative Cosmeceuticals—Non-woven Tissues as New Biodegradable Carriers." *Cosmetics* 8 (3): 65.

Moyer-Gusé, Emily, and Karyn Riddle. 2009. *The Media's Impact on Children: A Handbook for Parents, Educators, and Policymakers.* Lexington, KY: Aresta.

Mukta, S., and Friedman Adam. 2010. "Cosmeceuticals in Day-to-day Clinical Practice." *Journal of Drugs in Dermatology* 5: 62–66.

Müller-Wille, Staffan. 2006. "Linnaeus' Herbarium Cabinet: A Piece of Furniture and Its Function." *Endeavour* 30 (2): 60–64.

Murdoch, Walter. 1929. *The Making of Australia.* Melbourne: Whitcombe & Tombs Ltd.

Muzik, Otto, Tom J. Mangner, William R. Leonard, Ajay Kumar, and James G. Granneman. 2017. "Sympathetic Innervation of Cold-Activated Brown and White Fat in Lean Young Adults." *Journal of Nuclear Medicine* 58 (5): 799–806.

Narvaez-Chicaiza, Monica Andrea. 2020. "Harm Reduction Policies Where Drugs Constitute a Security Issue." *Health Care Analysis* 28 (4): 382–390.

Navarro, Roberto Campos, Edith Yesenia Peña Sánchez and Alfredo Paulo Maya. 2017. "Aproximación crítica a las políticas públicas en salud indígena, medicina tradicional e interculturalidad en México (1990–2016)." *Salud colectiva* 13: 443–455.

Nazarizadeh, Ali, Peyman Mikaili, Milad Moloudizargari, Shahin Aghajanshakeri, and Soheil Javaherypour. 2013. "Therapeutic Uses and Pharmacological Properties of *Plantago major* L. and its Active Constituents." *Journal of Basic and Applied Scientific Research* 3 (9): 212–221.

Newland, Amy Reigle, ed. 2005. *The Hotei Encyclopedia of Japanese Woodblock Prints*. Leiden: Hotei Publishing.

Neytendablaðið. 1 October 2013. "Made in Iceland."

Nguyen, Julie K., Natasha Masub, and Jared Jagdeo. 2020. "Bioactive Ingredients in Korean Cosmeceuticals: Trends and Research Evidence." *Journal of Cosmetic Dermatology* 19 (7): 1555–1569.

Nguyen, Ngoc Minh Duyen. 2021. "Factors influencing Finnish Generation Z Consumer Behaviors towards Green Purchase of Cosmetics." *Theseus*.

No, Yeon A., Eun Jung Ko, Sun Young Choi, Kwang Ho Yoo, Beom Joon Kim, and Myeung Nam Kim. 2015. "P002: An Anti-aging Effect of Cream Containing Mucus Secreted by Snails." 프로그램북 (구 초록집) 67 (2): 395.

Norðanfari. 16 June 1875.

Nordenfelt, Lennart. 1995. *On the Nature of Health: An Action-Theoretic Approach*. Dordrecht: Springer Science and Business Media.

Nova, Esther, Noemí Redondo-Useros, Rosa M. Martínez-García, Sonia Gómez-Martínez, Ligia E. Díaz-Prieto, and Ascensión Marcos. 2020. "Potential of Moringa oleifera to Improve Glucose Control for the Prevention of Diabetes and Related Metabolic Alterations: A Systematic Review of Animal and Human Studies." *Nutrients* 12 (7): 2050.

NTR. 2020. Official site.

Núñez Guillén, María Elena, José Artur da Silva Emim, Caden Souccar, and Antonio José Lapa. 1997. "Analgesic and anti-inflammatory activities of the aqueous extract of *Plantago major* L." *International Journal of Pharmacognosy* 35 (2): 99–104.

Nurdin, Muhammad Syafruddin, A. Imam, A. Thahir, and V. Hadju. 2018. "Supplementations on Pregnant Women and the Potential of *Moringa Oleifera* Supplement to Prevent Adverse Pregnancy Outcome." *International Journal of Science and Healthcare Research* 3 (1): 71–75.

Nurvia, Okta, and Budi Sarasati. 2020. "The Influence of Beauty Vloggers on Purchasing Decisions Involving Skin Care Products." *KnE Social Sciences*: 65–79.

O'Hagan, Andrew, and Connie Smith. 2017. "A New Beginning: An Overview of New Psychoactive Substances." *Forensic Research & Criminology International Journal* 5 (3): 00159.

Okorie, Chuku, Kola Ajibesin, Adekunle Sanyaolu, Adeena Islam, Selciya Lamech, Kudakwashe Mupepi, Tatenda Mupepi, Akeem Oseni, Oluwayemisi Oyeleke, and

Amos Abioye. 2019. "A Review of the Therapeutic Benefits of *Moringa Oleifera* in Controlling High Blood Pressure (Hypertension)." *Current Traditional Medicine* 5 (3): 232–245.

Oleg, Privalo, Glebova Ilona, Glinushkin Alexey, Sycheva Irina, Savchenko Ivan, and Kosolapov Vladimir. 2018. "Biological Activities of Derived Bioactive Components from Moringa Species: An Overview." *Entomology and Applied Science Letters* 5 (1): 82–87.

Önder, Mustafa. 2018. "Contribution of Plays and Toys to Children's Value Education." *Asian Journal of Education and Training* 4 (2): 146–149.

Oqaasileriffik – Sprogsekretariatet. 2005. *Peqqinnissaqarfinni taaguusersuutit Sundhedsvæsensterminologi.* Viborg: Nørhaven Book.

Ortiz de Montellano, Bernard. 1975. "Empirical Aztec Medicine." *Science* 188 (4185): 215–220.

O'Shaughnessy, Michael, and Jane Stadler. 2010. *Media and Society*. 5th ed. Melbourne: Oxford University Press.

Otten, Jennifer J., Karen Cheng, and Adam Drewnowski. 2015. "Infographics and Public Policy: Using Data Visualization to Convey Complex Information." *Health Affairs* 34 (11): 1901–1907.

Ouweneel, Arij. 2018. *Resilient Memories: Amerindian Cognitive Schemas in Latin American Art.* Columbus, OH: The Ohio State University Press.

Owens III, Frederick S., Oluwabunmi Dada, John W. Cyrus, Oreoluwa O. Adedoyin, and Georges Adunlin. 2020. "The Effects of Moringa Oleifera on Blood Glucose Levels: A Scoping Review of the Literature." *Complementary Therapies in Medicine* 50: 102362.

Pancaroğlu, Oya. 2001. "Socializing Medicine: Illustrations of the Kitāb al-Diryāq." *Muqarnas* 18: 155–172.

Park, Robert. 1998. "Size Counts: The Miniature Archaeology of Childhood in Inuit Societies." *Antiquity* 72 (276): 269–281.

Parnell, Jade. 2017. "Vlogging: A New Phenomenon, but is it a Concern for People's Health?" *Journal of Aesthetic Nursing* 6 (4): 196–198.

Passie, Torsten, and Simon Brandt. 2018. "Self-Experiments with Psychoactive Substances: A Historical Perspective." In *New Psychoactive Substances. Handbook of Experimental Pharmacology*, edited by Hans Maurer and Simon Brandt, 69–112. Cham: Springer.

Patnaik, Akankshya, Sushanta Tripathy, and Aishwarya Dash. 2021. "Identifying the Features Influencing Sustainable Products: A Study on Green Cosmetics." In *Advances in Mechanical Processing and Design*, 631–640. Springer: Singapore.

Peacock, Amy, Raimondo Bruno, Natasa Gisev, Louisa Degenhardt, Wayne Hall, Roumen Sedefov, Jason White, Kevin V. Thomas, Michael Farrell, and Paul Griffiths. 2019. "New Psychoactive Substances: Challenges for Drug Surveillance, Control, and Public Health Responses." *The Lancet* 394 (10209): 1668–1684.

Pearce-Duvet, Jessica. 2006. "The Origin of Human Pathogens: Evaluating the Role of Agriculture and Domestic Animals in the Evolution of Human Disease." *Biological Reviews* 81 (3): 369–382.

Peeren, Esther. 2017. "Perspective." In *Symptoms of the Planetary Condition: A Critical Vocabulary*, edited by Mercedes Bunz, Birgit Mara Kaiser, and Kathrin Thiele, 91–96. Lüneburg: Meson Press.

Peeren, Esther. 2020. "Enter through the Gift Shop: The Rural Pauper Colony of Veenhuizen as a Tourist Attraction." *Collateral* 23: d ISSN 2506-7982.

Peña-Lévano, Luis, Colton Adams, and Shaheer Burney. 2020. "Latin America's Superfood Economy." *Choices* 35 (4): 1–6.

Penix-Tadsen, Phillip. 2013. "Latin American Ludology: Why We Should Take Video Games Seriously (and When We Shouldn't)." *Latin American Research Review* 48 (1): 174–190.

Pernisch, Romana, Daniele Dell'Aglio, and Abraham Bernstein. 2021. "Beware of the Hierarchy—An Analysis of Ontology Evolution and the Materialisation Impact for Biomedical Ontologies." *Journal of Web Semantics* 70: 100658.

Petraškienė, Renata, Skaidra Valiukevičienė, and Jūratė Macijauskienė. 2016. "Associations of the Quality of Life and Psychoemotional State with Sociodemographic Factors in Patients with Psoriasis." *Medicina* 52 (4): 238–243.

Pétursson, Pétur. 17 June 1989. "Þá voru 6 menn á Íslandi syndir." *Morgunblaðið*.

Pflaeging, Jana, and Hartmut Stöckl. 2021. "Tracing The Shapes of Multimodal Rhetoric: Showing the Epistemic Powers of Visualization." *Visual Communication* 20 (30): 397–414.

Philip, Robert Kemp. 1864. *The Dictionary of Medical and Surgical Knowledge and Complete Practical Guide in Health and Disease for Families, Emigrants, and Colonists: By the Editor of the "Dictionary of Useful Knowledge"*. London: Houston and Wright.

Philips, Susan. 2001. "Gender Ideology: Cross-cultural Aspects." In *International Encyclopedia of the Social & Behavioral Sciences*, 6016–6020. London: Elsevier.

Pilling, Jayne, ed. 2012. *Animating the Unconscious: Desire, Sexuality and Animation.* New York: Wallflower Press.

Pitarakis, Brigitte. 2021. "Toys, Childhood, and Material Culture in Byzantium." In *Ludics: Play as Humanistic Inquiry*, edited by Rapti Vaassiliki and Eric Gordon, 243–276. Singapore: Palgrave Macmillan.

Pitt, Sarah, Cinzia Dedi, Pamela Taylor-Harris, M.A. Graham, and Alan Gunn. 2015. "Antimicrobial Properties of Mucus from the Brown Garden Snail Helix Aspersa." *British Journal of Biomedical Science* 72 (4): 174–181.

Pliny. 1906. *Natural History* 5.75.8. Digital version in the Packard Humanities Institute Latin Texts online, edited by K.F.T. Mayhoff, Naturalis Historiae, Bibliotheca scriptorum Graecorum et Romanorum Teubneriana, Lipsiae.

le Polain De Waroux, Yann, and Eric Lambin. 2013. "Niche Commodities and Rural Poverty Alleviation: Contextualizing the Contribution of Argan Oil to Rural Livelihoods in Morocco." *Annals of the Association of American Geographers* 103 (3): 589–607.

Poli, Roberto. 1996. "Ontology for Knowledge Organization." *Advances in Knowledge Organization* 5: 313–319.

Pop, Rebeka-Anna, Zsuzsa Săplăcan, and Mónika-Anetta Alt. 2020. "Social Media Goes Green—The Impact of Social Media on Green Cosmetics Purchase Motivation and Intention." *Information* 11 (9): 447.

Prichard, James Cowles. 1843. *The Natural History of Man; Comprising Inquiries into the Modifying Influence of Physical and Moral Agencies on the Different Tribes of the Human Family*. London: Moyes and Barclay.

Prioreschi, Plinio. 1996. *A History of Medicine*. Omaha: Horatius Press.

Quave, Cassandra Leah, Usha Lohani, Alonso Verde, José Fajardo, Diego Rivera, Concepción Obón, Arturo Valdes, and Andrea Pieroni. 2010. "A Comparative Assessment of Zootherapeutic Remedies From Selected Areas in Albania, Italy, Spain and Nepal." *Journal of Ethnobiology* 30 (1): 92–125.

Rábová, Tereza Klabíková. 2015. "Marketing Communication of SMEs Specialized in Cosmetic Industry in Magazines for Women." *Procedia-Social and Behavioral Sciences* 175: 48–57.

Racy, Ali Jihad. 2016. "Domesticating Otherness: The Snake Charmer in American Popular Culture." *Ethnomusicology* 60 (2): 197–232.

Radcliffe, Sarah, and Isabella M. Radhuber. 2020. "The Political Geographies of D/decolonization: Variegation and Decolonial Challenges of /in Geography." *Political Geography* 78: 102128.

Randolph, Whitney, and Kasisomayajula Viswanath. 2004. "Lessons Learned from Public Health Mass Media Campaigns: Marketing Health in a Crowded Media World." *Annual Review of Public Health* 25: 419–437.

Rasmussen, L., and J. Mercer. 2004. "A Comparison of Thermal Responses in Hands and Feet of Young and Elderly Subjects in Response to Local Cooling as Determined by Infrared Imaging." *Thermology International* 14: 71–76.

Rasoanaivo, Philippe, Alain Loiseau, Lucile Allorge-Boiteau, and Vinany Loharanombato. 2018. "Development and Commercialization of Asiaticoside in Madagascar." In *African Indigenous Medical Knowledge and Human Health*, edited by Charles Wambebe, 115–130. Boca Raton, FL: CRC Press.

Ravikumar, Thangaraj. 2012. "A Study on Impact of Visual Media Advertisements on Women Consumers Buying Behaviour in Chennai City." *International Journal of Multidisciplinary Research* 2 (2): 78–89.

Reich, Adam, Kalina Welz-Kubiak, and Łukasz Rams. 2014. "Apprehension of the Disease by Patients Suffering from Psoriasis." *Advances in Dermatology and Allergology / Postępy Dermatologii i Alergologii* 31 (5): 289.

Reihling, Hanspeter. 2008. "Bioprospecting the African Renaissance: The New Value of Muthi in South Africa." *Journal of Ethnobiology and Ethnomedicine* 4 (1): 9.

Reina, Elaine, Nouf Al-Shibani, Eman Allam, Karen S. Gregson, Michael Kowolik, and L. Jack Windsor. 2013. "The Effects of Plantago Major on the Activation of the Neutrophil Respiratory Burst." *Journal of Traditional and Complementary Medicine* 3 (4): 268–272.

Rentetzi, Maria. 2020. "The Epistemology of the Familiar: A Hymn to Pandora." In *Boxes: A Field Guide*, edited by Susane Bauer, Martina Schlünder, and Maria Rentetzi, 37–42. Manchester: Mattering Press.

Reutter, Louis. 1915. "Des remèdes d'origine humaine et animale prescrits au temps des Romains en Europe." *Revue d'Historie de la Pharmacie* 12: 179–180.

Reyes-Chilpa, Ricardo, Silvia Laura Guzmán-Gutiérrez, María Campos-Lara, Ezra Bejar, Helia Reyna Osuna-Fernández, and Griselda Hernández-Pasteur. 2021. "On the First Book of Medicinal Plants Written in the American Continent: *The Libellus Medicinalibus Indorum Herbis from Mexico*, 1552. A Review." *Boletín Latinoamericano y del Caribe de Plantas Medicinales y Aromáticas* 20 (1): 1–27.

Rhodes, Tim, Magdalena Harris, Francisco Gutiérrez Sanín, and Kari Lancaster. 2021. "Ecologies of Drug War and More-Than-Human Health: The Case of a Chemical at War with a Plant." *International Journal of Drug Policy* 89: 103067.

Richter, Tobias, Sascha Schroeder, and Britta Wöhrmann. 2009. "You Don't Have to Believe Everything You Read: Background Knowledge Permits Fast and Efficient Validation of Information." *Journal of Personality and Social Psychology* 96 (3): 538.

Rijksoverheid. 2021. Government of The Netherlands Official Website.

Roed, Murray, and Robert Fulton. 2011. *Okanagan Geology South: Geologic Highlights of the South Okanagan, British Columbia.* Kelowna: Okanagan Geology Committee Sandhill Book Marketing Ltd.

Rohini, Grace. 2002. "Cosmeceuticals: Functional food for the Skin." *Natural Foods Merchandiser* 23: 92–99.

Rooney, Anne. 2013. *The History of Medicine.* New York: Arcturus.

Rosengren, Izabella. 2020. "The Women who Make Argan Oil Want Better Pay." *BBC*, February 6, 2020.

Rosse, Cornelius, and José Mejino. 2003. "A Reference Ontology for Biomedical Informatics: The Foundational Model of Anatomy." *Journal of Biomedical Informatics* 36 (6): 478–500.

Roy, Hélène. 2017. "El inca y su refugio mítico: Espacio de regeneración y de resistencia." *Diálogo andino* 54: 103–111.

Rummel, Rudolph Joseph. 1994. *Death by Government.* New Brunswick-London: Transaction Publishers.

Russell, Richard, Aurélie Porcheron, Jennifer R. Sweda, Alex L. Jones, Emmanuelle Mauger, and Frederique Morizot. 2016. "Facial Contrast is a Cue for Perceiving Health from the Face." *Journal of Experimental Psychology: Human Perception and Performance* 42 (9): 1354.

RÚV. 2021. "Ísland enn langefst á lista yfir losun á hvern íbúa." August 20, 2021.

Sabina, María, and Eunice V. Pike (Trans.). 1957. *Album Insert. Mushroom Ceremony of the Mazatec Indians of Mexico. María Sabina.* New York: Folkways Records Album No. FR8975.

Sabovljević, Marko S., Aneta D. Sabovljević, Nur Kusaira K. Ikram, Anantha Peramuna, Hansol Bae, and Henrik T. Simonsen. 2016. "Bryophytes – An Emerging Source for Herbal Remedies and Chemical Production." *Plant Genetic Resources* 14 (4): 314–327.

Sagona, Antonio. 2018. *The Archaeology of the Caucasus: From Earliest Settlements to the Iron Age.* New York: Cambridge University Press.

Sahagún, Bernardino De. 1577. *General History of the Things of New Spain by Fray Bernardino de Sahagún: The Florentine Codex.*

Sahagún, Bernardino De, Creator. 1577. *General History of the Things of New Spain by Fray Bernardino de Sahagún: The Florentine Codex. Book XI: Natural Things.* Pdf. Retrieved from the Library of Congress.

Sahagún, Bernardino De. 1999. Reprint. *La Historia General de las Cosas de Nueva España.* Mishawaka: Porrua.

Sahay, Surbhi, Upasana Yadav, and Sheetal Srinivasamurthy. 2017. "Potential of *Moringa oleifera* as a Functional Food Ingredient: A Review." *International Journal of Food Science and Nutrition* 2 (5): 31–37.

Saheed, Sabiu, Ajani E. Oladipipo, Abubakar A. Abdulazeez, Sulyman A. Olarewaju, Nurain O. Ismaila, Irondi A. Emmanuel, Quadri D. Fatimah, and Abubakar Y. Aisha. 2015. "Toxicological Evaluations of *Stigma maydis* (corn silk) Aqueous Extract on Hematological and Lipid Parameters in Wistar Rats." *Toxicology Reports* 2: 638–644.

Sanabria, Emilia. 2021. "Vegetative Value: Promissory Horizons of Therapeutic Innovation in The Global Circulation of Ayahuasca." *Biosocieties* 16: 387–410.

Sarkar, Rashmi, Shikha Chugh, and Shivani Bansal. 2016. "General Measures and Quality of Life Issues in Psoriasis." *Indian Dermatology Online Journal* 7 (6): 481.

Sarpur: Menningarsögulegt gagnasafn. 2021. "Sundkennsla." February 4, 2021.

Schaffer, Simon. 2009. "The Asiatic Englighenments of British Astronomy." *The Brokered World: Go-Betweens and Global Intelligence, 1770–1820*, edited by Simon Schaffer, Lissa Roberts, Kapil Raj, and James Delbourgo, 49–104. Sagamore Beach: Watson Publishing.

Schemmel, Matthias. 2012. "The Transmission of Scientific Knowledge from Europe to China in the Early Modern Period." In *The Globalization of Knowledge in History*, edited by Jürgen Renn, 269–293. Berlin: Open Access.

Schemmel, Matthias. 2020. "Global History of Science as a Knowledge Resource for the Anthropocene." *Global Sustainability* 3 (e22): 1–8.

Schendel, Gordon. 2021. "Aztec Herbs and Therapies." In *Medicine in Mexico: From Aztec Herbs to Betatrons*, 62–73. New York, NY: University of Texas Press.

Schiebinger, Londa. 2004. *Plants and Empire.* London: Harvard University Press.

Schiebinger, Londa. 2017. *Secret Cures of Slaves: People, Plants, and Medicine in The Eighteenth-Century Atlantic World.* Stanford, CA: Stanford University Press.

Schooley, Janine, Christine Mundt, Pascale Wagner, Judith Fullerton, and Mark O'Donnell. 2009. "Factors Influencing Health Care-Seeking Behaviours among Mayan Women in Guatemala." *Midwifery* 25 (4): 411–421.

Seddon, Toby. 2009. *A History of Drugs: Drugs and Freedom in the Liberal Age.* London: Routledge-Cavendish.

Seelig, Michelle. 2019. "Popularizing the Environment in Modern Media." *The Communication Review* 22 (1): 45–83.

Seggiaro, Luis. 1969. *Medicina Indígena de America.* Buenos Aires: Editorial Universitaria de Buenos Aires.

Semedo, Maria Guilherme, Ana Leonor Pereira, and João Rui Pita. 2021. "The Influence of German Science on Cinchona and Quinine Research in Portugal in the

Second Half of the 19th Century." *Die Pharmazie-An International Journal of Pharmaceutical Sciences* 76 (8): 396–402.

Seo, Yuri, Angela Gracia Cruz, and 'Ilaisaane ME Fifita. 2020. "Cultural Globalization and Young Korean Women's Acculturative Labor: K-beauty as Hegemonic Hybridity." *International Journal of Cultural Studies* 23 (4): 600–618.

Sera-Shriar, Efram. 2015. "Human History and Deep Time in Nineteenth-century British Sciences: An Introduction." *Studies in History and Philosophy of Science Part C: Studies in History and Philosophy of Biological and Biomedical Sciences* 51: 19–22.

Sessa, Ben. 2018. "The 21st Century Psychedelic Renaissance: Heroic Steps Forward on the Back of an Elephant." *Psychopharmacology* 235 (2): 551–560.

Shafeai, Reza, and Shadie Sijanivandi. 2019. "The Impact of Celebrity's Promotion Considering the Self-Concept Mediator Role on the Attitude of Consumers Women Cosmetic in Tehran City." *Quarterly Journal of Brand Management* 6 (1): 141–186.

Sharma, Andrew. 2017. "Multiculturalism, Diversity and Stereotypes: Engaging Students with Images in Media." *Media Watch* 8 (1): 20–29.

Sharma, Meghna, Prachi Trivedi, and Jimnee Deka. 2021. "A Paradigm Shift in Consumer Behaviour towards Green Cosmetics: An Empirical Study." *International Journal of Green Economics* 15 (1): 1–19.

Sheina, Elena, Elena Smirnova, and Irina Ryabkova. 2017. "The Developmental Potential of Toys and Games." In *The Routledge International Handbook of Early Childhood Play*, edited by Tina Bruce, Pentti Hakkarainen, and Milda Bredikyte, 305–312. London: Routledge.

Shevchuk, Nikolai, and Sasa Radoja. 2007. "Possible Stimulation of Anti-tumor Immunity using Repeated Cold Stress: A Hypothesis." *Infectious Agents and Cancer* 2 (1): 1–9.

Shigeru, Oikawa. 2005. "The Maintenance of Tradition in the Face of Contemporary Demands: A Reassessment of Meiji Prints." In *The Hotei Encyclopedia of Japanese Woodblock Prints*, edited by Amy Reigle Newland, Volume 1, 261–265. Amsterdam: Hotei Publishing.

Shin, Kyu-Ok, and Hang-Sik Park. 2019. "Antiaging Cosmeceuticals in Korea and Open Innovation in the Era of the 4th Industrial Revolution: From Research to Business." *Sustainability* 11 (3): 898.

Sigurðsson, Sigurður. 1976. "Um berklaveiki á Íslandi." *Læknablaðið* 62: 3–50.

Siipi, Helena. 2008. "Dimensions of Naturalness." *Ethics and the Environment* 13 (1): 71–103.

Siipi, Helena. 2020. "Food, Food Substitutes and Food Supplements [Special Issue]." *Argumenta* 5 (2): 247–260.

Silva, Ana, Manuel José Fonseca, Paulo Ribeiro Cardoso, Maria Castro Fonseca, and Andreia Teixeira. 2021. "Factors Influencing the Purchase Intention of Cruelty-Free Cosmetics in Portuguese Consumers–An Exploratory Approach." *International Conference on Information Technology & Systems*, 256–268. Cham : Springer.

Silva, Luciana, Valeria Valim, Ana Paula C. Pessanha, Leda M. Oliveira, Samira Myamoto, Anamaria Jones, and Jamil Natour. 2008. "Hydrotherapy Versus

Conventional Land-based Exercise for the Management of Patients with Osteoarthritis of the Knee: A Randomized Clinical Trial." *Physical Therapy* 88 (1): 12–21.
Singer, Peter. 1997. "Neither Human nor Natural: Ethics and Feral Animals." *Reproduction, Fertility and Development* 9 (1): 157–162.
Singh, Devendra, and Dorian Singh. 2011. "Shape and Significance of Feminine Beauty: An Evolutionary Perspective." *Sex Roles* 64 (9): 723–731.
Singhal, Aakanksha, and Garima Malik. 2021. "The Attitude and Purchasing of Female Consumers Towards Green Marketing Related to Cosmetic Industry." *Journal of Science and Technology Policy Management* 12 (3): 514–531.
Simkin, John. 2020. "Alexander Apsit." *Spartacus Educational.*
Sivasankarapillai, Vishnu Sankar, Reshmi Madhu Kumar Nair, Abbas Rahdar, Simona Bungau, Dana Carmen Zaha, Lotfi Aleya, and Delia Mirela Tit. 2020. "Overview of the Anticancer Activity of Withaferin A, an Active Constituent of the Indian Ginseng Withania somnifera." *Environmental Science and Pollution Research* 27: 26025–26035.
Six, Jean-François. 1998. *Thérèse De Lisieux. Son Combat Spirituel, Sa Voie*. Paris: Éditions Du Seuil.
Skaltsa, Elena. 2015. *Ιστορια Τησ Φαρμακευτικησ*. Athens: Kallipos.
Sklair, Leslie, ed. 2020. *The Anthropocene in Global Media: Neutralizing the Risk.* London-New York: Routledge.
Smith, Barry. 2012. "Ontology." In *The Furniture of the World: Essays in Ontology and Metaphysics*, edited by Guillermo Hurtado, and Oscar Nudler, 47–68. Leiden: Brill.
Smith, Rosanna K., Elham Yazdani, Pengyuan Wang, Saber Soleymani, and Lan Anh N. Ton. 2021. "The Cost of Looking Natural: Why the No-makeup Movement May Fail to Discourage Cosmetic Use." *Journal of the Academy of Marketing Science* 50 (2): 324–337.
Smithsonian Institution Archives. 2014. Accession 14-196, Smithsonian Institution, Website Records.
Soens, Tim, Raf De Bont, and Maïka De Keyzer. 2020. "At the Edge of Resilience: Making Sense of COVID-19 from the Perspective of Environmental History." *Journal for the History of Environment and Society* 5: 9–20.
Solianik, Rima, Albertas Skurvydas, Astra Vitkauskienė, and Marius Brazaitis. 2014. "Gender-Specific Cold Responses Induce a Similar Body-Cooling Rate but Different Neuroendocrine and Immune Responses." *Cryobiology* 69 (1): 26–33.
Soloaga Díaz, Paloma, and Carlos Muñiz Muriel. 2011. "La publicidad de moda de lujo: efectos en la autopercepción de mujeres españolas." *Indumenta: Revista del Museo del Traje* 2: 106–122.
Soto Laveaga, Gabriela. 2009. *Jungle Laboratories*: *Mexican Peasants, National Projects, and the Making of the Pill.* Durham: Duke University Press.
Steininger, Rita. 2008. *Indianen.* Aartselaar: Deltas.
Stephens, John. 2002. *Ways of Being Male: Representing Masculinities in Children's Literature and Film.* New York: Routledge.
Stewart, Susan. 2017. *Painted Faces: A Colourful History of Cosmetics.* Gloucestershire: Amberley Publishing Limited.

Suh, Soyoung/ 서소영. 2018. "Marketing Medicine to Koreans." In *Imagining Chinese Medicine*, edited by Vivienne Lo and Penelope Barrett, 467–478. Leiden - Boston: Brill.

Sullivan, Nikki. 2006. "Transmogrification: (Un)Becoming Others." *The Transgender Studies Reader*, edited by Susan Stryker and Stephen Whittle, 552–564. New York: Routledge.

Sultana, Ashiqha. 2021. "Impact of Online Advertising and the Use of Cosmetic Products: A Study on the Influence of Online Advertisements and Change in the Purchasing Behaviour of Women in Kerala." *International Journal of Communication and Society* 3 (2): 112–119.

Sutelman, Pablo, Gemma Vilahur, Laura Casani, and Lina Badimon. 2020. "The Role of Nutritional Additives in Prevention: Dietary Supplementation with Spirulina Reduces Myocardial Damage and Improves Cardiac Function Post-myocardial Infarction in Swine." *European Heart Journal* 41 (2): ehaa946–2973.

Swift, R. W. 1932. "The Effects of Low Environmental Temperature upon Metabolism: II. The Influence of Shivering, Subcutaneous Fat, and Skin Temperature on Heat Production." *The Journal of Nutrition* 5 (3): 227–249.

Stadford, Patrycja. 2015. *Angielskie słwka dla dzieci.* Poznan: Publicat.

Szendy, Peter. 2019. *The Supermarket of the Visible*. New York: Fordham University Press.

Tamang, Sapan, Manjil Gupta, and Kishore Kumar Thapa. 2019. "Cinchona Plantation in Darjeeling Hills: History and Extension." *Indian Science Cruiser* 33 (6): 57–60.

Tarlov, Alvin. 1996. "Social Determinants of Health: The Socio-Biological Translation." In *Health and Social Organization*, edited by David Blane, Eric Brunner, and Richard Wilkinson, 71–93. London: Routledge.

Tashbayeva, Kadicha. 2001. *Petrogliphs of Central Asia* [sic]. Bishkek: International Institute for Central Asian Studies of Samarkand.

Tettey, Justice, Conor Crean, Susan C. Ifeagwu, and Martin Raithelhuber. 2018. "Emergence, Diversity, and Control of New Psychoactive Substances: A Global Perspective." In *New Psychoactive Substances*, edited by Hans H. Maurer, Simon D. Brandt, 51–67. Cham: Springer.

Tewary, Tavishi, Ashish Gupta, Vaibhav Mishra, and Jitender Kumar. 2021. "Young Working Women's Purchase Intention Towards Organic Cosmetic Products." *International Journal of Economics and Business Research* 22 (2–3): 256–277.

Thukaram, Maithreyi. 2019. "A Green Thumbs-Up for the Future of Cosmetics." *Chemical Engineering Progress* 115 (10): 56.

Tipton, Mike J. 1989 (1979). "The Initial Responses to Cold-water Immersion in Man." *Clinical Science* 77 (6): 581–588.

Torshin, Ivan. 2007. *Physiology and Medicine.* New York: Nova Science.

Tsafrir, Jenni, and Avi Ohry. 2001. "Medical Illustration: From Caves to Cyberspace." *Health Information & Libraries Journal* 18 (2): 99–109.

Tsoutsos, Dimosthenis, Despoina Kakagia, and Konstantinos Tamparopoulos. 2009. "The Efficacy of Helix Aspersa Müller Extract in the Healing of Partial Thickness

Burns: A Novel Treatment for Open Burn Management Protocols." *Journal of Dermatological Treatment* 20 (4): 219–222.

Tucker, Arthur O., and Jules Janick. 2019. *Flora of the Voynich Codex: An Exploration of Aztec Plants.* Cham: Springer Nature.

Tupper, Kenneth. 2008. "The Globalization of Ayahuasca: Harm, Reduction or Benefit Maximization?" *International Journal of Drug Policy* 19 (4): 297–303.

Türel, Idris, Hanefi Özbek, Remzi Erten, Ahmet Cihat Öner, Nureddin Cengiz, and Orhan Yilmaz. 2009. "Hepatoprotective and Anti-inflammatory Activities of *Plantago major* L." *Indian Journal of Pharmacology* 41 (3): 120.

Umhverfisstofnun. 2019. *Sund- og baðstaðir: Handbók.* Reykjavik: Umhverfisstofnun.

Urrutia Gómez, Andrea Carolina. 2015. "El lápiz labial: Identidad, presentación y experiencias de la feminidad en Lima, Perú." *Fronteras* 2 (1): 21–48.

Valerio, Luis. 2005. "Toxicological Aspects of the South American Herbs Cat's Claw (*Uncaria tomentosa*) and Maca (*Lepidium meyenii*)." *Toxicological Reviews* 24 (1): 1–35.

Van Groesen, Michiel. 2012. *The Representations of the Overseas World in the De Bry Collection of Voyages (1590–1634).* Leiden-Boston: Brill.

Venkatapuram, Sridhar. 2013. *Health Justice: An Argument from the Capabilities Approach.* New York, NY: John Wiley & Sons.

Voultsiadou, Eleni. 2010. "Therapeutic Properties and Uses of Marine Invertebrates in the Ancient Greek World and Early Byzantium." *Journal of Ethnopharmacology* 130 (2): 237–247.

Wafer, Lionel. 1699. *A New Voyage Amp Descripition of the Isthmus of America.* Oxford: Hakluyt Society.

Waimitila, K. W. 2009. *Kamusi ya Picha.* Nairobi: Vide-Muwa.

Wallis, Robert J. 2019. "Art and Shamanism: From Cave Painting to the White Cube." *Religions* 10 (1): 54.

Wang, B., ed. 2003. *Huang di nei jing* (Huangdi's internal classics, 206 BC–AD 24). Publishing House of Ancient Chinese Medical Books, Beijing.

Wang, Jordan V., Evan A. Rieder, Elizabeth Schoenberg, Christopher B. Zachary, and Nazanin Saedi. 2020. "Patient Perception of Beauty on Social Media: Professional and Bioethical Obligations in Esthetics." *Journal of Cosmetic Dermatology* 19 (5): 1129–1130.

Wang, Lei, and Jin Hwa Lee. 2021. "The Impact of K-beauty Social Media Influencers, Sponsorship, and Product Exposure on Consumer Acceptance of New Products." *Fashion and Textiles* 8 (1): 1–29.

Wells, Paul, Johnny Hardstaff, and Darryl Clifton. 2008. *Re-imagining Animation: The Changing Face of the Moving Image.* Lausanne: Ava Book.

Wen, Xinyi. 25 April 2022. "The Doctrine of Signatures in Early Modern Medicine." Paper presented at British Society for the History of Pharmacy.

Westerhoff, Jan. 2005. *Ontological Categories.* Norfolk: Oxford University Press.

Wilk, Richard. 2006. *Home Cooking in the Global Village: Caribbean Food from Buccaneers to Ecotourists.* London: Berg.

Wilk, Richard. 2007. "'Real Belizean Food': Building Local Identity in the Transnational Caribbean." In *Food and Culture: A Reader*, edited by Carole Counihan and Penny Van Esterik, 2nd edition, 244–255. New York: Routledge.

Wilkinson, Lise. 1992. *Animals and Disease: An Introduction to the History of Comparative Medicine.* Cambridge: Cambridge University Press.

Winkelman, Michael, and Michael Winkelman. 2019. "Archeological Investigations of Ancient Psychoactive Substances." *Journal of Psychedelic Studies* 3: 261–263.

Wolski, Grzegorz J., Beata Sadowska, Marek Fol, Anna Podsędek, Dominika Kajszczak, and Agnieszka Kobylińska. 2021. "Cytotoxicity, Antimicrobial and Antioxidant Activities of Mosses Obtained from Open Habitats." *PloS One* 16 (9): e0257479.

Wood, David. 2006. "Indigenismo and the Avant-garde: Jorge Sanjinés' Early Films and the National Project." *Bulletin of Latin American Research* 25 (1): 63–82.

Wood, John George. 1868. *The Natural History of Man: Being an Account of the Manners and Customs of the Uncivilized Races of Men. Africa.* London: George Routledge and Sons.

Wood, John George. 1870. *The Natural History of Man: Being an Account of the Manners and Customs of the Uncivilized Races of Men. Australia, New Zealand, Polynesia, America, Asia, and Ancient Europe.* London: George Routledge and Sons.

Wood, Theodore. 1890. *The Rev. J.G.Wood: His Life and Work.* Cambridge: Cambridge University Press.

Woods, Abigail, Michael Bresalier, Angela Cassidy, and Rachel Mason Dentinger. 2018. *Animals and the Shaping of Modern Medicine.* Cham: Palgrave Macmillan.

Wu, Yi, Sandra Mulkens, and Jessica M. Alleva. 2022. "Body Image and Acceptance of Cosmetic Surgery in China and the Netherlands: A Qualitative Study on Cultural Differences and Similarities." *Body Image* 40: 30–49.

Xu, Zhen, Tahir Islam, Xiaobei Liang, Naeem Akhtar, and Mohsin Shahzad. 2021. "'I'm Like You, and I Like What You Like': Sustainable Food Purchase Influenced by Vloggers: A Moderated Serial-Mediation Model." *Journal of Retailing and Consumer Services* 63: 102737.

Yahya, Abdul-Halim, Gun-Hean Chong, and Chin-Ping Tan. 2014. "The Phytochemical Properties of a New Citrus Hybrid (Citrus Hystrix × Citrus Microcarpa)." *Scienceasia: Journal of the Science Society of Thailand* 40 (2): 121–124.

Yang, Hui-Ju, and Kuo-Chia Yang. 2015. "Impact of Psoriasis on Quality of Life in Taiwan." *Dermatologica Sinica* 33 (3): 146–150.

Yardley, Christopher. 2015. *The Representations of Science and Scientists on Postage Stamps.* Canberra: Australian National University Press.

Yinka Déné Language Institute. 2018. Main Website.

Yuan, Lingyan, Zhitong Bing, Jiani Han, Xiaoli An, Xingkui Liu, Rui Li, Caiyun Wang, Xueqiang Sun, Lei Yang, and Kehu Yang. 2020. "Study on The Anti-Tumor Mechanism Related to Immune Microenvironment of *Bombyx Batryticatus* on Viral And Non-Viral Infections of Hepatocellular Carcinoma." *Biomedicine and Pharmacotherapy* 124: 109838.

Zahidul, Islam, S. M. Rashadul Islam, Faruk Hossen, Kazi Mahtab-ul-Islam, Md. Rakibul Hasan, and Rezaul Karim. 2021. "Moringa oleifera is a Prominent Source of Nutrients with Potential Health Benefits." *International Journal of Food Science* Article ID 6627265.

Zapata, Félix, José Manuel Matey, Gemma Montalvo, and Carmen García-Ruiz. 2021. "Chemical Classification of New Psychoactive Substances (NPS)." *Microchemical Journal* 163: 105877.

Zhang, Yi, Chunfang Wang, Chenxia Liu, Xiao Wang, Bingjie Chen, LianMou Yao, Yongjin Qiao, and Hongjian Zheng. 2020. "Recent Developments in *Stigma Maydis* Polysaccharides: Isolation, Structural Characteristics, Biological Activities and Industrial Application." *International Journal of Biological Macromolecules* 150: 246–252.

Zhaychybekov, B. 2012. *Кыргызско- русско- английский словарик для детей в картинках.* Kutaalam: Bishkek.

Zhoh, Choon-Koo, Min-Hee Lee, In-Young Kim, and Ji-Young Shin. 2016. "Skin Improvement Effect of Mask Pack with Snail Fermented Extract." *Journal of the Korean Applied Science and Technology* 33 (1): 30–40.

Zurlo, Joanne, Deborah Rudacille, and Alan M. Goldberg. 1994. *Animals and Alternatives in Testing: History, Science, and Ethics.* New York: Mary Ann Liebert.

Þjóðviljinn. 31 October 1891. "Sundkennsla í Reykjanesinu 1891."

Þórðarson, Sveinn. 1998. *Saga hitaveitna og jarðhitanýtingar á Íslandi.* Safn til iðnsögu Íslendinga Volume XII. Reykjavik: Hið íslenzka bókmenntafélag.

FILMOGRAPHY

Burke, Marie, director. 2005. *Spirit Doctors.*

Gómez, Ana, and Paola Gómez, directors. 2020. *Rujotay k'aslemal / La vida retoñando a través de la salud.*

Limousin, Fabien. 2021. *Nawak.*

Index

Note: Page numbers in *italics* refer pages with figures and tables.

About the Author

Milton Fernando Gonzalez Rodriguez earned his PhD at the University of Amsterdam in 2019, having previously been affiliated with the University of Iceland and Malmö University. In 2021, he joined the Cultural History since 1750 Team, KU Leuven, as a Marie Skłodowska-Curie Fellow. The focus of his work lies on how everyday objects, artifacts, and rituals encode/produce knowledge and how they can be used to obtain data on the set of attitudes, beliefs, and assumptions societies have about themselves, O/others, their surroundings, and the natural world. Fernando is interested in how external characterizations deploy images and words at an epistemic, ontological, and cultural level. In his current project, *Remedial Nature: Medicinal Efficacy in Images and Words since the Advent of Mass Media in Western Europe* (EU Horizon 2020, Grant Agreement 101026198), he explores how representations, materialized in health-enhancing consumables, have been mobilized historically and linguistically to imply a relation between nature, medicinal efficacy, (peripheral) identities, and alternative (un)scientific knowledge(s). In 2022 and 2023, Fernando will be a Visiting Scholar at the Department of History and Philosophy of Science (University of Cambridge) and Leibniz Institute for Educational Media | Georg Eckert Institute (Leibniz Association). His forthcoming publications include the monographs *Indigeneity in Latin American Cinema* (2022) and *Ontologies and Natures: Knowledge about Health in Visual Culture* (2022).

www.ingramcontent.com/pod-product-compliance
Ingram Content Group UK Ltd.
Pitfield, Milton Keynes, MK11 3LW, UK
UKHW041452071026
15587UKWH00010B/823

9 781666 909494